RED LIGHT THERAPY

THE COMPLETE GUIDE TO TREATING FAT LOSS, ANTI-AGING, MUSCLE GAIN, HAIR LOSS, SKIN DAMAGE AND BRAIN IMPROVEMENT WITH RED LIGHT THERAPY

BY: RAPHAEL MERRILL

© Copyright 2019 by Raphael Merrill
All rights reserved.

This document is geared towards providing exact and reliable information with regards to the topic and issue covered. The publication is sold with the idea that the publisher is not required to render accounting, officially permitted, or otherwise, qualified services. If advice is necessary, legal or professional, a practiced individual in the profession should be ordered.

- From a Declaration of Principles which was accepted and approved equally by a Committee of the American Bar Association and a Committee of Publishers and Associations.

In no way is it legal to reproduce, duplicate, or transmit any part of this document in either electronic means or in printed format. Recording of this publication is strictly prohibited and any storage of this document is not allowed unless with written permission from the publisher. All rights reserved.

The information provided herein is stated to be truthful and consistent, in that any liability, in terms of inattention or otherwise, by any usage or abuse of any policies, processes, or directions contained within is the solitary and utter responsibility of the recipient reader. Under no circumstances will any legal responsibility or blame be held against the publisher for any reparation, damages, or monetary loss due to the information herein, either directly or indirectly.

Respective authors own all copyrights not held by the publisher.

The information herein is offered for informational purposes solely, and is universal as so. The presentation of the information is without contract or any type of guarantee assurance.

The trademarks that are used are without any consent, and the publication of the trademark is without permission or backing by the trademark owner. All trademarks and brands within this book are for clarifying purposes only and are the owned by the owners themselves, not affiliated with this document.

TABLE OF CONTENTS

Introduction 1

Chapter 1 2

What Is Red Light Therapy? 2

    Research And Historical Timeline Of Red Light Therapy 2

    How Does Red Light Therapy Work? 7

    How Is Red Light Therapy Used? 11

    Red Light Therapy Application 15

    Benefits Of Red Light Therapy 19

    What Do I Go For Red Light Therapy? 25

    Possible Side Effect And Risk Of Red Light Therapy 27

Chapter 2 30

Red Liht Therapy For Specific Purposes 30

    Red Light Therapy For Weight Loss 30

    Red Liht Therapy For Baldnes And Hair Growth ... 36

    Treating Inflammation And Pain With Near Infrared And Red Light Therapy 45

    Red Light Therapy For Knee And Osteoarthritis 57

    Red Light Therapy For Wrist And Hand Pain 59

    Red Light Therapy For Spine Discomfort 60

    Bottom Line: Red Light Therapy Is An Important Natural Cure For Arthritis And Joint Pain 62

Chapter 3 64

Choosing A Red Light Therapy Device 64

    Top 5 Overall Lights 92

Chapter 4 104

Red Light Dosing 104

    How To Use Your Red / Near Infrared Light System 111

Chapter Five 127

Frequently Asked Questions About Red Light Therapy 127

Conclusion 175

INTRODUCTION

You likely must have seen an uptick in red-light, luxury fitness class advertisements lately peppering your Instagram feed. Or maybe it is the horror film-segue masks in plastic face that celebrities like Chrissy Teigen and Jessica Alba have flaunted to tip you towards the emerging trend of red light. If you wonder what red light therapy is exactly, how it works and if you can benefit from adding it to your spa routine, join me as we take a wonderful tour of the light and learn more about this fresh, warm treatment in this book.

CHAPTER 1

WHAT IS RED LIGHT THERAPY?

Red light therapy uses a red light that penetrates wavelengths directly through the skin of a patient. This is a painless, chemical-free process that does not produce heat so that the light emitted does not trigger any discomfort if the surface epidermis comes into contact. During the treatment process, low red light levels are absorbed in the skin at a depth of approximately 6-10 millimeters. Red light therapy trials have shown that it can be used for the treatment of several medicinal foods and cosmetic disorders in the fields of neurology, physical therapy, and dermatology as a successful non-drug treatment technique.

Research and Historical Timeline of Red Light Therapy

Over the years, the use of red light therapy has been developed through the work and experiences of scientists all over the world. Although a relative' newcomer' in the Eastern Medicine community, the roots of light therapy can be traced back to ancient times. It was the Greeks who realized first that exposure to light created healing properties that might aid in restoring health.

In the early 1800s, the Danish scientist Dr Niels Finsen was awarded the Nobel Peace Award for his efforts to demonstrate the positive effects of wavelengths in tuberculosis treatment.

In the 1960s, European researchers found that certain single wavelengths have a significant therapeutic effect on tissue treatment through a photo-stimulation system. A good example of photo stimulation would be the use of light for the treatment of newborns with jaundice, a common liver condition that causes the skin and eyes of a baby to yellow.

A scientist named Endre Mester from Budapest made a major discovery on the results of treatment with low power ruby laser in the late1960s, not long after the first functioning laser was invented. Like other scientists of his era, Mester tried to use a high-performance laser to kill malignant tumors. Under the skin of laboratory rats, he implanted tumor cells and placed them in a personalized light. To his dismay, doses believed to be high-power laser energy did not destroy the tumor cells. Rather, he found that the skin incisions made to insert abnormal cells tended in treated animals to heal more quickly compared to incisions of non-lighterly control animals. The low-power light rather stimulated the skin to heal more quickly. Mester was one of the first researchers to discover how mitochondrial chromophores absorb photons in cells of the skin and how stem cell activation allows improved tissue repair and cure. The therapeutic value of red light was discovered in his research; it was investigated how different wavelengths of light can promote skin, muscle, nerve, tendon, cartilage, bone healing and also denture and periodontal tissues. It was Mester's initial work that eventually led to the development in mono-chromatic light treatment for ongoing medical research-for which he became a photo-biomodulation father.

Almost ahead of the1990s, NASA scientists developed pioneering technologies using red lighting for space missions. More extensive research originally used to promote plant growth in the surroundings of spacecraft has shown that using red light penetrated deep into the tissues not only can stimulate cell growth, but can facilitate both human and animal cures.

Red light was then examined to find out whether RLT could increase the energy inside humans ' cells for its potential application in medicine. The scientists hoped that RLT could be an effective way to treat the weightlessness of muscle atrophy, slow wound healing, and problems of bone density during space travel.

You may also have heard of Red Light Therapy (RLT) by other names including:

- Photobiomodulation (PBM)
- Low Level Light Therapy (LLT)
- Soft Laser Therapy
- Cold Laser Therapy
- Biostimulation
- Low-Powered Laser Therapy.

Red light therapy is believed to be photodynamic therapy when used with photosensitizing drugs. In this type of therapy, light is used only as a drug activator.

Several different types of red light therapy are available. Red-light beds in salons, including stretch marks and wrinkles, are said to help reduce cosmetic skin issues. Red light therapy in the doctor can be used to treat more severe conditions such as psoriasis, slow-healing wounds and even chemotherapy adverse events.

While there is considerable evidence that RLT can be an effective remedy for certain disorders, there is somewhat an excellent deal to be learned about how it works.

How Does Red Light Therapy Work?

Light therapy has been shown to provide strong therapeutic benefits for the living tissue in our bodies for over 30 years. It is well understood that our bodies require light; without it physiological and emotional changes would occur and that vitamin D would be seriously deficient. Human bodies usually have different reactions to light, but light energy can move through human tissues much better than other wavelengths with red-light therapy in the region of 600–900 nm. Once the wavelength of red light is penetrated and absorbed into the skin, it converts cellular energy, not only activating our body's naturally occurring processes but kick-start' some metabolic events which include the following:

- Formation of new capillaries
- Increased energy level as a result of ATP production
- Increases the blood flow / circulation, providing more oxygen and tissue resources to our cells and tissues
- Decreases or stimulates inflammation
- Increased production of collagen and fibroblasts
- Activates the lymphatic system.
- Enhances DNA or RNA synthesis
- Cellular clean up or increased phagocytosis.
- Repair and restoration of the damaged soft connective tissue
- Decreasing oxidative / free radical damage, which is linked to many effects of aging.

When the energy from light is absorbed into our species, especially within the range of 600 nm-900 nm, research shows that biological responses can be generated. These rejuvenating, stimulating' energy boosts ' allow the cells to perform their natural functions at an increased level. Red light therapy affecting all skin layers may touch blood cells, lymph nodes, nerves and hair follicles, depending on the body part of the red light projected. The physiological responses to light therapy can also be seen in red.

Leanne Venier, a renowned engineer, scientist and expert in light frequencies, and the healing effects of color therapy, says that, because of its effects on humans, red light naturally attracts attention, energizes, stimulates and' represents their survival, joy, and passion.' Besides being noticed, the colored red also induces a "fight or flight" reaction, which accelerates circulation, causes our heart to hit faster, increases the production of sweat glands, and increases our stress levels.

Although the color red may not be so pleasant, it can be of benefit to the healing process, as these particular wavelengths of red light produce a biochemical reaction in our cells that enhances mitochondrial function. Much like the sun's UV rays that damage our skin, red light therapy will stimulate our body's natural defense system. Sunburn, freckles, and tanning are also significant. It also has the remarkable power to reactivate complex nutrient processes in our bodies that can help to rejuvenate or heal.

Red light is thought to work in cells that stimulate mitochondria by creating a biochemical effect. Mitochondria are the cell's powerhouse— this is the source of the cell's fuel. ATP (adenosine triphosphate) is the energy molecule found in the cells of all living organisms.

By increasing the mitochondrial function with RLT, a cell may produce additional ATP. Cells can work more effectively, rejuvenate, and restore damage with more fuel.

RLT is different from laser or IPL treatments because it does not affect the surface of the skin. Laser and pulsed light treatments operate by causing controlled damage to the outer skin surface, which then contributes to the reparation of tissue. RLT circumvents this harsh step by directly stimulating skin regeneration. The light from RLT penetrates approximately 5 millimeters under the surface of the skin.

How Is Red Light Therapy Used?

Hundreds of clinical studies and thousands of lab studies have been performed since the initial experiments in space to determine whether RLT has medical benefits.

Several studies have shown promising results, but the effects of red light therapy are still controversial. For instance, the Center-for Medicare-and-Medicaid-Services (CMS) has concluded that there are insufficient evidences to show that such devices are better than currently existing injury, ulcer, and pain treatment services.

Further clinical research is needed to further demonstrate the effectiveness of Red Light

Therapy. There is currently some evidence that shows RLT is beneficial. The benefits include the following:

- Promotes hair growth in individuals with androgenic alopecia
- Promotes tissue repair and wound healing
- Helps to treat carpal tunnel syndrome for a short time
- Facilitates the treatment of slow-healing wounds, such as diabetic foot ulcers
- Reduces lesions of the inflammation and relief of psoriasis
- Short-term treatment of pain and discomfort
- Minimizes some side effects of cancer treatment, such as mucositis
- Helps in mending sun damage
- Enhances the buildup of collagen to improve skin complexion and diminish wrinkles
- Prevent reoccurring cold sores from herpes

- Relieves inflammation and pain in people with Achilles tendons problem
- Help in diminishing scars
- Improves the health of joints in individual with degenerative osteoarthritis

Red light therapy is not covered or endorsed by insurance bodies for these conditions as a result of sufficient evidence. Nevertheless, several insurance companies now reimburse the use of RLT to avoid oral mucositis when treating cancer.

While the Internet is often flooded with reports of miraculous cures for almost any health condition, red light therapy is definitely not all about it. For most circumstances, RLT is considered experimental.

Red lighting therapies have been shown to do the following:

- Treating depression, postpartum depression, and seasonal disorder

- Enhances the lymphatic system to help "detoxify" the body
- Boosting the immune system
- Reducing cellulite
- Weight loss aids
- Treating pain in the back or neck
- Fights periodontitis and dental infection
- Healing Acne
- Treating cancer

Additional light therapies were used to help with some of the above conditions. For example, studies have found that white light therapy is more effective than red light in treating depression symptoms. Blue light treatment of limited effectiveness is more widely used for acne.

Similar Treatment Alternative

Red light wavelengths are not the only clinical wavelengths to be investigated. Similar experiments were performed in animals, including blue light, green light and a combination of different wavelengths.

Other light-based therapies are available. Ask your doctor about:

- Laser therapies
- Natural sunlight
- Blue or green light therapy
- Ultraviolet light therapy B (UVB)
- Sauna Light therapy
- Psoralen and ultraviolet lighting A (PVA)

Red Light Therapy Application

Since red light therapy helps in speeding up skin cure, it may be used to solve a number of issues including:

- *Inflamed Acne Marks and Acne:* However, Red light therapy is not used in killing acne-causing bacteria but it will help in minimizing the inflammation effects caused by the acne. Infrared and Red lights penetrate the skin at various levels and enable the cells to rebuild the body. It repairs acne-destroying skin tissues. This leads to quicker acne healing and prevents further tissue damage which can lead to acne cells. Blue Light Therapy, on the other hand, has been clinically proven to kill P. acne bacteria, which are the commonest cause of acne.

- *Bites:* Due to the red light, the potential to improve healing, bite wounds or punctures in the skin will be healed quicker as the blood flow to the region increases.
- *Bruises:* These are caused either by direct trauma or by damaged capillaries by bleeding to the skin tissues. Because the blood can \not leave the body without any skin separation, it produces a bluish hue which is what we also call an inflammation. Red light therapy will be able to supply the region with nutrient-rich blood more

efficiently, helping to rebuild and form new capillaries.

- *Mild Burns:* Red Light Therapy does not release heat and will not do further damage caused by burns. What it will do is to improve the area's blood supply, so that our organism's normal protection and repair mechanism can do its job more efficiently.

- *Cuts, Scraping, and Wound Care:* As mentioned, increased blood flow to the area helps speed up the ability of the body to repair itself naturally.

- *Dry Skin and Psoriasis:* The Red Light penetrates the skin thickened and enhances the skin cells. As the surface of the skin is handled with increased blood flow, more nutrients are distributed to this region. It ensures that the appetite of the body is quenched and nurtured. Blood flows oxygen-rich to the treated areas and also improves hydration caused by good blood supply.

- *Scars and Stretch Marks*: Stretch marks are caused, whether by weight loss or age, by saggy skin. Body collagen depletion leads to a thin, stretched and saggy body. Red light therapy helps to stimulate the production of collagen and thus prevents further development of stretch marks. It also tends to lighten and reduce bruises and even skin color overall.
- *Sun Damage:* Red light is a superstar when sun damage is corrected. UV-free LED lamps are used to provide red light therapy safely and effectively. The red wavelength of light spurs cellular activity to prevent damage to the sun. It can lighten spots with age.
- *Wrinkles:* Folds start to creep on our face (or neck), due to loss of collagen. Red light therapy helps to promote the development of collagen and fibroblasts to help correct these

dumb signs of aging. It works under eye wrinkles, wrinkles of the forehead, laughs, and crowing feet.

Benefits of Red Light Therapy

1. Healing wounds, tissue repair, and pain relief

Light-emitting diode technology (LED) provides drugs a device capable of providing light deep into the body's tissues at a higher wavelength (600-1000 nm deeper penetration) optimally to heal wounds, minimize pain and repair tissues. Many basic biological mechanisms may explain the impact of RLT concerning wound healing.

- Higher light density can promote stimulation in the skin by increasing cell growth, migration and adherence
- Light therapy can influence skin cells through the regeneration of fibroblasts, keratinocytes and immune cell modulation

- Increasing cytokine-signal molecules that encourage cells to move to sites of inflammation, infection and trauma.
- Stimulating growth factors such as inflammation, proliferation, homeostasis, and tissue restructuring which aids different stages of wound healing.

2. *Hair loss and Anti-aging effects*

Red light therapy has become increasingly popular due to its ability to stimulate, repair, and enhance the facial skin appearance. The circulation and fibroblastic activity, collagen production, and healing are promoted during RLT treatments. This influence has provided a positive result, along with decreased skin roughness, wrinkles, and fine lines, with increased collagen densities, enhanced skin tone, texture, and sound of the teeth. Clinical and research trials have shown that red light treatment is successful in several skin conditions, such as rosacea and acne.

Alopecia (hair loss) is a chronic disorder that affects over half of the world's population. The most common type of androgenic alopecia affects 50% of men over the age of 40 and 75% of women over the age of 65. Although controversial about its ability to reverse balding effect, controlled clinical trials have shown that RLT can enhance hair growth in both men and women by stimulating hair follicle epidermal stem cells and moving the Follicle into anagen phase (This is a stage hair enters a state of proper and active growth).

3. Improving joint and muscle health

LLLT has been used clinically for patients with arthritis as a short-term relief treatment for pain and morning stiffness since the late 1980s. Now an FDA-approved treatment, doctors use it to assist chronic joint pain patients. The ability of red light therapy to promote the development of collagen, rejuvenate cells, increase blood flow and regeneration of cartilage makes this an active healing tool for the root causes of osteoarthritis, rheumatoid arthritis and many other inflammatory joint problems. The range 800-900 nm appears to be optimum for penetration of the wavelength (to arthritic joints) and about 820 nm for maximum cellular effects. The clinical studies indicate that red light therapy works because it can easily reduce inflammation in the joints, which often decreases discomfort almost immediately after treatment.

Light therapy is pain-free andnon-invasive, making it popular with animals such as horses and home pets.

4. *Light therapy can also improve the health of the muscles*

According to a study in Lasers Med Science, in several experimental models of skeletal muscle damage and repair, positive results with LLLT have been published. We have myosatellite cells in our bodies, a type of muscle stem cell that is actively involved in growth and repair. These cells normally exist in a relaxed, inactive state, but they become fully functional muscle cells in the cure process when penetrated by LLLT. Stimulation of myosatellite cells plays an important role in the regeneration of skeletal muscle in response to injury or exercise trauma.

5. Minimize side effects of cancer treatments

NASA-technology has come a long way since it first experimented with red light therapy to improve plant life in shuttle missions. In recent years, NASA has taken advantage of new level of lighting therapy when scientists develop HEALS, a high emissivity aluminum light substratum, which involves using far-red / near-infrared light-emitting diode devices that release long wavelength energy as photons. HEALS has successfully stimulated cells to assist in recovery while at the same time reducing debilitating side effects from chemotherapy and radiation therapies for bone marrow and stem cell transplant. NASA has carried out a two-year clinical trial with cancer patients, HEALS, for the treatment of a widespread and extremely painful side-effect of cancer therapies called oral mucositis, in collaboration with the University of Alabama at Birmingham Hospital. The study concluded that 96 percent of patients had reduced pain due to HEALS. In addition to the effectiveness of this procedure, researchers have improved HEALS technology for clinical use, especially in patients with pediatric brain tumors and those suffering from hard to heal wounds or infections such as diabetic skin ulcers that cause severe burns.

6. *Helps Fatigue and Depression*

In clinical researches, continued exposure to red light therapy has proved effective for people suffering from depression or fatigue in clinical studies. Research shows that, when red light wavelengths enter the facial skin, neurons start an increasing production of neurotransmitters that raises the mood. Treatment in patients who have been moderately depressed, tired or suffering from SAD (seasonal affective disorder) has reported a more joyful, energized, and positive feeling.

In particular, how it interacts with the mechanism of action in acupuncture administration. Eastern doctors think that light is an energy form and that light therapy depends on the belief that colors are correlated with body chakra. Such chakras (electrical energy centers throughout the body) are expected to have a profound effect on our emotions and our mood. Light therapy penetrates deep into the tissues rather than using needles to stimulate light energy in chakra zones or meridian points. The technique allows for connections in our bodies; red light therapy can help to improve our physical, spiritual, and emotional well-being by activating these points all over the body.

What Do I Go For Red Light Therapy?

While traditional doctors in the western world still view the use of red light therapy as an alternative therapy, it has been used widely in East Asia and Russia for many years. While eastern medicine is less stringent on government approval, most western doctors in the West still claim that insufficient evidence supports its efficacy for all patients, even though many of the Federal Pharmaceutical Administration's Red Light Therapies (FDA) have been approved.

Most people who are interested in LLLT therapies have the opportunity to ask your primary care provider or the chiropractor to refer you to a dermatologist, oncologist, orthopedist and rheumatologist or neurologist who administers red light therapy.

A popular option for those who want red-light therapy skin benefits is a visit to a spa, salon, or gym that offers roughly $500 per session. Nevertheless, if you choose this option, a trained and qualified physician will administer the care you receive. Today, some products also manufacture red light therapy for home use. Home red light therapy treatments such as Trophy Skin's Rejuvalite, the DPL Revive II and the Photon Therapy System of

Norlanya tend to have good reviews of their efficacy in the treatment of dermatological conditions. For many people, these devices may be more affordable for ongoing sessions as prices range from $50 for a small mobile unit to $800 for a deluxe model. As with any red light therapy system that you buy, you should always take care, know the danger and above all consult your doctor before beginning your home therapy.

Most gyms now sell body-wide red light therapy beds. Make sure that you choose this option to ask whether the wavelengths are between 620 nm and 800 nm. You should also check whether the beds in the gym were FDA approved as a precautionary measure.

It is important to note that because red light therapy is still considered an "experimental" treatment; many insurance policies generally do not cover it.

Possible Side Effect and Risk of Red Light Therapy

Red Light Therapy is a safe, non-evasive well-tolerated treatment is considered to be red light therapy. It is mostly unlikely that an individual will have any side effects. Nonetheless, some mild and short term cases have been reported, such as eye strain, dizziness, headache, vomiting, sleep disturbance and irritability. While all these negative side effects are generally considered acceptable, it may help you eliminate or minimize any pain that arises by cutting back your prescription duration, shortening the length of your sessions, adjusting the period you receive your treatments or taking longer breaks between sessions.

You should always consult with a doctor before treatment to prevent any risk and/or side effects when using red light therapy. The optimal dosage and timing of the red light can be calculated by a doctor to reduce the potential of negative side effects-Safety measures for your eyes should be taken as your facial skin gloves and specially designed coverings are the best safety guards if you use red light therapy.

Like any medicine you get, you should always talk to your doctor and report any drug or counter-medications that you take.

CHAPTER 2

RED LIGHT THERAPY FOR SPECIFIC PURPOSES

RED LIGHT THERAPY FOR WEIGHT LOSS

Being excessively over-weight is something that can lead to a variety of other diseases, including blood pressure, diabetes, backaches, arthritis, asthma etc.

While losing weight is vital for the overall health of your body, it is equally important that the method of weight loss is safe and does not have any side effects. One of the most advanced technologies for weight loss is red light therapy.

Red light therapy is considered to be one of the very effective slimming procedures. It is a safe method without needles, incisions or operations. The red light therapy works by stimulating the mitochondria in the fat cell nucleus, which releases fatty acids into the space between them. Extra fatty acids are then excreted and urinated from the skin. This process is so simple and natural.

The system is also useful when burning more than 500 calories per session. By using this technology, over 2000 more calories can be used regularly than a normal person who does not use this therapy. This is an innovative system that works with an extremely simple method that securely consumes the calories.

How Does Weight Loss Red Light Therapy Works?

RLT works on a very simple mechanism that I describe in two main areas, bio-energetics and blood flow.

- *Bio-energetics:* Red light therapy essentially activates the fat cell's mitochondria.

Mitochondria, also known as the cell leader, increases glucose oxidation when activated. This is because of the wavelength of red light between 600 nm and 1000 nm, which activates a central copper enzyme in our cells. Therefore, more cellular energy is produced, and more glucose is efficiently consumed. It reduces stress and leads to healthy cells. The metabolic rate increase ultimately leads to fat loss.

- *Blood flow* -Moreover, red light therapy in the area where it drops is believed to boost blood flow. It produces a large amount of energy in the cells and increases blood flow. Better blood flow contributes to a healthy body supply of essential nutrients.

Safe without Any Side Effects

Unlike other slimming treatments, such as surgery and other risky methods, this treatment is intended to provide benefits without damaging the body.

While the fat in the tissue under your skin is healthy, it clearly affects your waistline.

It is a painless method that removes centimeters from your body's target areas. This makes your body slimmer and slimmer. This tightens the loose skin and colors this. The greatest benefit is that it allows the patient to function throughout the procedure and does not require any recovery time. And the best results followed.

Red Light Therapy Benefits For weight loss

One of the major reasons for weight loss using this therapy is that it reduces the appetite of the patient. Less appetite means that a person will not eat more, and the additional fat will not accumulate. At the same time, the body uses the stored fat. Red light therapy also affects fat and contributes to local and systemic loss of it. Within days, you lose several inches to make your appearance smarter and healthier.

The obvious goal of this therapy is to lose weight, but it also increases the energy level of the body. During this procedure one remains highly active and energized. This protects lean tissue and is extremely non-invasive.

In addition to losing weight, which is the obvious advantage, photobiomodulation eliminates inches from your target area. It also stimulates and tones loose skin, but various clinical studies support these claims while it is used. This is where the term "contouring body" is derived.

The advantage of this procedure is that you can undergo the medication at home if you have the device. This does not impede your routine, and while the treatment is ongoing, you can continue with your daily tasks.

RLT also has a significant benefit of increasing energy levels due to increased metabolism and blood flow, and more energy is equivalent to better health.

With a variety of weight loss products and ideas sold in the market which often lead to side effects, something we have discussed above can be easily skeptical. It should be remembered, however, that this is a totally safe procedure. In order to let you know if it has any side effects, I have explained it below.

Are There any side effects of weight loss With Red Light?

Red light therapy is a non-invasive technology and has never caused any type of side effects. Patients have never complained of any discomfort or of any side effects during treatment. The red light used is modulated and drains and reduces the fat cells. In addition, new collagen and elastin are added to tighten and tone the skin and make it look young and beautiful. Red light therapy works absolute wonders when you are completely healthy and slim.

There are lots of researches in this area and over the years scientists have studied and tested this technique. Red light therapy is known to be a safe and effective way to lose weight and restore skin sensation and smoothness.

RED LIHT THERAPY FOR BALDNES AND HAIR GROWTH

Red light therapy is a safe, efficient and natural treatment for hair loss which becomes more common with professionals and the public. Supported by a strong foundation of peer-reviewed clinical research, red light therapy has increased hair count and hair density for both men and women. Besides being a natural baldness cure for both genders, laboratory studies have shown that it can even help restore dog coats and other mammals. And all these benefits come without negative side effects.

A review of the work on red light therapy and hair regeneration is discussed in this section. Write about the science and its effect on baldness behind natural light.

How Red Light Therapy Assist in Treating Hair Loss

The short version is this: A LED light therapy system provides healthy, concentrated wavelengths of natural light to your skin without toxins, UV ray or unnecessary energy. This red and close infrared light wavelength activate mitochondria element in your cells similar to natural sunlight, minimize oxidative stress and increase circulation, helping you to create more core energy to power your body.

Having power more effective in your entire body enhances physical function, accelerates the healing process and decreases inflammation and pain, as many peer-reviewed studies have shown. It also activates the dermal papilla cells, which play a significant role in hair cycling and growth regulation.

Red Light Research Shows Is an Effective Natural Hair Loss Treatment

Hair loss is one of the most common consequences of the aging of more than half of the world's population. Over 50% of men over the age of 40 have Androgenetic Alopecia or severe hair loss. Seventy-five percent of women over 65 also have alopecia.

Fortunately, red light therapy provides a safe and natural way to prevent hair loss and reverse it. It is supported by numerous clinical studies, trials, and meta-analyzes reviewed by peers.

Eight clinical studies, comprising a total of 11 randomized controlled double blind trials, were examined in a 2019 meta-analysis. Quantitative analysis showed that the hair density of people treated with red light therapy increased significantly. Hair growth has increased significantly with red light treatment over null and placebo.

Red Light Therapy More Effective Than Hair Growth Products with No Side Effects

Recent developments in non-surgical hair loss treatment have been evaluated in 2018 meta-analysis. Twenty-two studies were conducted by comparing red light therapy to other common therapies, such as hormone-regulatory drugs like Finasteride and Dutasteride. Importantly, while many of the medications studied had negative side effects in this meta-analysis, there was no red light therapy.

Red Light Increased Hair Count, Density, Thickness and Strength

Another 2017 meta-analysis analyzed 11 trials and 680 patients who received red light therapy for hair growth. Researchers noted important hair count and hair density changes. Furthermore, hair thickness and tensile strength have also been improved with natural light. People were asked about their encounters who were treated with red light and generally responded very favorably to treatments.

Red Light Effective for Male Pattern Baldness versus Fake Treatment

Researchers performed a six-month randomized double-blind study in a single study in 2018 with both red light therapy and a fake system. For 100 participants, one side of each participant's head received real red light therapy 3 times a week and the other side received placebo treatment. At the end of the trial, the red light therapy side was significantly higher than the placebo treating side. Hair thickness, hair count and hair re-growth have also improved significantly. Researchers found that red light therapy is an active, safe and well-tolerated treatment for baldness of the male pattern.

Treating Male Baldness Treatment

In 2019, researchers conducted a six-month study examining men with pattern hair loss and protein expression changes in their dermal papilla tissue, which are responsible for hair growth. Over 6 months, participants are held every other day for 25 minutes of red light therapy. Through analyzing which proteins are up-regulated, researchers have concluded that red light therapy promotes hair growth and reverses the cycle of balding through the enhancement of the function of dermal papilla.

An additional study was conducted in 2014 to determine the safety and physiological effects of red light treatment on men with pattern baldness. 44 people had a scalp segment trimmed to a height of 3 mm. The area has been photographed and tattooed. One team was punished with red light every other day for 16 weeks, while the second was treated with guilt. After the study, researchers found:

- Significant increase in hair count post-treatment in the Red Light treatment group
- No adverse or side effects were reported
- 35 percentage increase in hair growth in the Red Light group
-

Treating Female Pattern Baldness with the Red Light Therapy

Ten (10) years ago, there were limited possibilities for female hair loss solutions. In the past decade, more attention has been paid to women's pattern hair loss, which has contributed to many research and treatment methods. Red light therapy is currently one of women's most proven and tested hair loss treatments.

One researcher who performed the above experiment on men decided to recreate it for female participants with hair loss, to test the effectiveness of red light therapy in women with normal hair loss. The double-blind, randomized trial was done in the same way: the area of 47 female participants was reduced to 3 mm by their scalp. The area was photographed and tattooed. One team was treated with red light every other day for 16 weeks, while the second was treated with a hoax. Upon completion of the test, researchers showed even better results on hair growth for women than men:

- Significant increase in post-treatment hair growth for women

- No adverse or side effects were reported
- 37% rise in the red light treatment group hair growth

Red Light Therapy and Topical work well together: A 2017 review looked at the effects of red light therapy and topical ointment (Minoxidil 5%) In the sample, 45 people were split into 3 groups: red light therapy, topical ointment and a combination group. Researchers concluded that treatments for red light therapy are successful. Scientists have suggested the use of both red and topical light to promote hair regrowth.

51% Increase In Women's Hair Growths: another 2017 study studied the effect of red light therapy on women with hair loss. The Ludwig-Savin Baldness scale was used by researchers to evaluate hair loss in women. They found that the number of women who received red light therapy at 650 nm increased 51 percent.

Studies Show Widespread Hair Growth use for Red Light

A wide range of other hair growth benefits have also been shown by numerous lab studies. Here is a quick grasp at some of the studies reviewed:

- *Hair growth for alopecia dogs:* 7 alopecia dogs of various ages, breeds and sexes, have been diagnosed with red light therapy. At the end of the study, the growth of coat regrowth in each animal was improved and significantly improved in six out of seven animals.
- *Hair cunts in various mammal:* Animals treated with red light therapy experienced 60 percent hair growth in comparison with 42 percent of untreated animals. Red-light animals also display a much longer hair than untreated mammals.

Promising results Treating Lichen Planopilaris

Lichen planopilaris is a form of scarring hair loss which occurs when a common skin disease, a lichen planus, affects skin areas where hair is present. This condition tends to be gradual and only 10 percent of the most effective therapies respond. Lichen Planus is an inflammatory disease and the normal anti-inflammatory treatment of red light is well known.

While further studies are needed, this trial in 2017 is a successful beginning. Eight patients with lichen planopilaris are treated for 15 minutes a day, for 6 months with red light therapy. The results were good.

- Enhanced hair thickness after 3 and 6 months
- Erythema reduced, or less patchy and reddened skin
- Lichen planopilaris disease activity decreased

TREATING INFLAMMATION AND PAIN WITH NEAR INFRARED and RED LIGHT THERAPY

The inflammation, particularly chronic inflammation, of millions of Americans has pain and physical function has decreased. A definition of inflammation is available here: forms, causes, symptoms and treatments. First, we explore clinical research and the potential for chronic inflammation treatment by red-light therapy, a natural cure that does not have most anti-inflammatory drugs ' distressing side effects.

What is inflammation?

Inflammation is not only a symptom, but in every living thing a complex process. Inflammation can be seen in your body as a conditioned response to danger. This is one of the first actions of an infection, germs, inflammation and cell damage in your immune system.

Causes

Injuries and wounds, fractures, splinters, and burns are obvious physical causes. Biological factors such as germ infection and stress also lead to inflammation. Chemical irritants, toxins, and alcohol can also cause inflammation. Environmental conditions can also affect the body, for example, bad sleep, poor food, malnutrition and prolonged exposure to blue light and radiation. These environmental factors may have a role to play in chronic inflammation.

Millions of Americans have inflammation-reducing pain and physical function, particularly chronic inflammation. The article provides a summary of inflammation: forms, causes, symptoms, and treatments. We also research the ability to treat chronic inflammation with red-light therapy, a natural remedy with many anti-inflammatory medicines which have no distressing side effects.

Symptoms and symptoms

Heat, redness, swelling, pain and loss of control are five common inflammatory signs. The pain is caused by chemicals like bradykinin and histamine, which trigger the body to activate nerve endings as a risk warning. There is also clinical evidence that depression and inflammation are associated with both depressive and suicidal inflammation.

Chronic or acute?

It's not all negative inflammation. In reality, acute inflammation helps our body recover from a crisis. Within a few hours, inflammation takes place in normal reaction, the pathogens are eliminated, and the repair process begins and then goes away. Recurrent and recurrent, acute inflammation, viral infections, allergic responses and foreign bodies are often caused by chronic inflammation. It can be very unpleasant and can worsen certain disorders, including gum disease, fever, arthritis and certain cancers.

Inflammation Pharmaceutical Drugs, Health Risks, and Side Effects

Inflammations are usually treated with NSAID or non-steroid anti-inflammatory medicinal products. These include lower risk, over and above pain counter forms such as aspirin and ibuprofen. People often take NSAIDs to treat more severe chronic inflammation. NSAIDs are also known as "Cox-2 inhibitors." Unfortunately, NSAIDs have an unpleasant past and a lengthy list of possible side effects and risks to the health.

The benefits of NSAIDs for people over 60 are usually higher. Despite all this, many doctors and patients try more natural inflammation and pain therapies that do not rely on potentially dangerous drugs.

Treatment of Inflammation with LED Light Therapy

The promise of natural red and near-infrared light therapy is enormous: natural inflammation therapy without the risks of conventional NSAIDs approved for use.

As discussed previously, light therapy provides the skin and cells with free, bright natural light. These red and near-infrared wavelengths activate these cells to produce more energy for the body. This reduces oxidative stress. As many peer reviews have shown, it improves function, heals rate, and decreases inflammation and pain.

Natural light treatment and inflammatory therapy: Red light therapy reduces chronic inflammation through increased blood circulation to infected tissue and has been shown in several clinical trials to enhance body antioxidant protection.

Dr. Michael Hamblin of the Harvard Medical School and the Massachusetts General Hospital is one of the world's foremost experts in photo-medicine. He investigated long-term light therapy and found that "one of its most reproducible effects is a reduction in inflammation that is particularly important when treating joint wounds, traumatic injuries, lung disorders, and brain disorders." Dr. Hamblin said that natural red and close wavelengths are "a very mild form of pressure that stimulates c defense mechanisms."

Dr. Hamblin states that natural red and near-infrared light wavelengths are "a very mild form of pressure which triggers defensive mechanisms in cells, for example when long wavelengths or clearly red light enters the body, Mitochondria shifts towards more power-efficient energy production and stimulates the development of anti-inflammatory or disease-fighting antioxidants."

- *Pain relief and post-surgery inflammation:* Researchers found that the post-op pain and swellings of patients treated with natural light therapy were decreased further, concluding that natural light therapy "is effective in reducing pain severity and inflammation after surgery."
- *Decreased oral inflammation:* Another recent study tested the ability of light therapy to reduce inflammation in periodontal cells in the mouth in highly inflammatory diseases. Researchers concluded that "the research has shown [light therapy] prevents inflammation caused by E endotoxins.
- *Muscles, exercise & soreness:* Numerous other tests examined the ability of light therapy to treat muscle soreness and

inflammation and pain related to exercise. A research in 2008 showed that natural light had a beneficial effect on muscle soreness symptoms. In a 2010 Brazilian study, people using light therapy before exercising eventually experienced less pain and inflammation following training.

- *Laboratory work on mammals:* The above-mentioned study aligns with previous studies of inflammatory markers in laboratory rats, which reliably show that therapies for light therapy boost muscle soreness and reduce inflammation.

Health & Fitness Leaders Suggest Light Therapy for Inflammation

The medical result shows that natural light can play a large part in treating inflammation and pain without the harmful side-effects of NSAID drugs. Additionally, some doctors and health and fitness experts explored their own performance in the treatment of inflammation and pain.

The following are samplings:

- *Dr. Sarah Ballantyne (aka Paleo Mom):* She biophysicist and best-selling author of the New York Times, Dr. Sarah spoke about her struggles with fibromyalgia joint pain and inflammation. After a year of use of a Joovv light therapy device, she declared,

    "I owe my current level of energy to my Joovv and my lack of joint pain... my own experience matches that documented in the scientific literature. The use of Joovv has resulted especially in enhanced strength, significant pain relief, improved mood, and I feel and look a lot younger"

- *World-famous trainers:* Jorge Cruise is a world-famous trainer and best-selling health & fitness writer. He clarified that his clients often have no proper exercise due to inflammation and joint pain. He has therefore introduced light therapy from

Joovv for himself and his clients to help overcome the suffering and now swears.
- Another world-renowned trainer, Ben Greenfield, says Light Therapy is a game-changer that helps competitors overcome the stress and inflammatory pain of exhausting workouts. Ben wrote a very useful light therapy guide on how it works for him and how to select the best device for you.

The findings of these prominent trainers and their clients are consistent with the results from the clinical research on the positive effect of light therapy on muscle tissue pain and inflammation.

Near Infrared and Red Light Proven to Minimize Joint Pain and reduce Arthritis Pain

Light has proven to reduce joint pain and alleviation of arthritis and other joint problems affect over 50 million American adults. The resulting pain has long been the first cause of injury in the nation and is usually handled with treatment and service.

The broad base of clinical research on natural-treatment arthritis–red light therapy (including photobiomodulation or PMB) –will be discussed here. Researches all over the world have discovered that red and near-infrared light has an important effect on joint pain reduction and increasing function & movement for people with arthritis. Every year more optimistic studies appear, and we will summarize a number below.

Arthritis in America

There are more than 100 forms it poses and different ways it starts among those 50 million Americans with arthritis. The bottom line, though, is pain and inflammation in most people with arthritis — painful, swollen joints that impair their mobility, health and chips ' quality of life over the years. Many types of arthritis may become remission if the person follows advice on medical treatments and lifestyle. Nevertheless, there is no treatment for arthritis in traditional medicine. The best chance is typically to manage the illness through pharmaceutical and/or surgical treatments. Doctors can, in some cases, also prescribe natural treatments such as vitamins, minerals and spices, acupuncture, electrical stimulation and hot and cold therapy.

There has been some peer reviewed clinical research showing that red and infrared light wavelengths have an important and positive impact on arthritis symptoms, such as joint pain and inflammation, by targeting the cell sources of this worsening disorder.

Red light therapy has been well established across hundreds of studies in the last three decades, with positive effects on arthritis, joint pain and inflammation. This is a brief survey of important results for osteoarthritis and rheumatoid arthritis along with wrist, arm, knee and spinal pain.

RED LIGHT THERAPY FOR KNEE AND OSTEOARTHRITIS

Several studies on red light therapy and knee osteoarthritis specifically are conducted. More are always coming out. In 2018, the authors of one study found that "reducing discomfort and increasing physical mobility after three months of stretching plus[red light] therapy" showed that two independent Brazilian studies concluded that a red light therapy plus exercise and stretching had significantly greater effect on the treatment of osteo-related knee pain than stretches or exercise alone..Researchers have concluded that patient knees "were decreased pains and increased physical activity after 3 months of stretching plus [red light] therapy."

- *Osteoarthritis Knee Pain:* Some other researches in major journals have since 2015 found a significant reduction of knee pain attributable to osteoarthritis by natural red light therapy.

- *Improved Range of Motion:* Recent studies of knee pain have shown that red light therapy not only decreases knee pain but also improves mobility and motion.
- *Cartilage Regeneration:* A study conducted in Lasers in Medical Science study, 2017 reveals that knee cartilage has been assessed in animal studies and red light has found that it significantly reduces pains and improves knee cartilage regeneration through "biochemical changes."
- *Treating Meniscus Tears:* European researchers carried out a double-blind, placebo-controlled trial in 2013 on pain levels in meniscal (meniscus tears) patients. Those researchers concluded:

"The treatment with light Therapy was associated with a substantial reduction in the number of symptoms compared with the placebo group: it should be seen in patients with meniscal tears who do not wish to undergo any surgical procedure."

- *General Knee Pain:* red light improves all joint issues that are not related to arthritis. However, systematic review in The Australian Physiotherapy Journal reviewed 11 light therapy clinical trials for chronic knee joint disorders. Light therapy decreased pain and improved overall joint function in all these trials.

RED LIGHT THERAPY FOR WRIST AND HAND PAIN

- *Hand Osteoarthritis in Women:* A 2015 systematic review of lasers in the medical sciences found that red light and ultrasound therapy showed strong results for the treatment of hand osteoarthritis for women, with a significant decrease in pain. In addition, this meta-analysis has recorded extensive and positive results for light therapy in knees, shoulders, back, jaws and other areas of arthritis.

- *Heberden's and Bouchard's Nodes in the Hand:*In a German study published in Lasers in Surgical Medicine, Bouchard's & Heberden's Nodes in hand examined 34 people with the sound outgrowth and swelling conditions known as the nodes of Bouchard & Heberden. Light therapy has been found "substantially reduced discomfort & ring and increased range of motions" and "very broad results."

RED LIGHT THERAPY FOR SPINE DISCOMFORT

Recent research has also shown ability to relieve spinal joint pain from conditions such as ankylosing spondylitis. A European research in 2016 found that red-light therapy and relaxation exercises combined reduced back pain more effectively than placebo-based therapy with Ankylosing Spondylitis (ABS) treatment.

Emerging Research Shows Light Therapy Can Treat Root Causes of Arthritis

Conventional medicine can treat symptoms of arthritis but provides no cure. Emerging laboratory work in 2018 shows that red light therapy can treat cellular arthritis and address the root cause.

Photo-medicine researchers in Brazil published a study in late 2018 that showed that red light therapy reduced all levels of cytokine after therapy and increased mammalian immune population. Researchers found: "Our results indicate that light therapy may change the inflammatory course of arthritis, accelerating its resolution through photobiostimulation of immune cells."

Years of Positive Study on Red Therapy and Arthritis

In recent years, several successful red-light therapies and arthritis studies have been based on positive conclusions from past research findings.

A systematic review of the Journal of Rheumatology found significant findings in 13 randomized controlled trials of arthritis performed prior to 2000:

- Rheumatoid Arthritis: Best results were shown in people with rheumatoid arthritis, while light therapy decreased their pain by 70% compared with placebo.
- Morning rigidity: Red light therapy reduced the morning rigidity of the participants by 27.5 minutes and significantly increased the mobility of the hand.

Bottom Line: Red Light Therapy Is an Important Natural Cure for Arthritis And Joint Pain

The world's study has shown a significant positive impact on red light therapy on arthritis, joint pain, inflammation and related symptoms. If you are having difficulty with arthritic joint pain and are looking for a natural therapy to treat pain and sorrow, you should definitely bear that in mind.

CHAPTER 3

CHOOSING A RED LIGHT THERAPY DEVICE

A wide range of options and variables can be very hard to sort for red light therapies by newcomers. In this post, we make sense to choose a red light therapy system and break down the key factors. And these factors include the following:

- Size & scope
- Design
- Safety
- Power
- Service

The most important factors of Red Light therapy are the service size and coverage. To achieve the best results, you need a bigger tool that can cover more of the body on a wider surface. A full-body operation with a larger system is safer and more effective than treating just a tiny part of your body.

More cells throughout your body are exposed to natural light with a larger device to increase the total transfer of energy. Some devices offer only targeted treatments but advertise complete coverage. Whether they are too low or bulky, like showerheads or belts, you have to change your body or system constantly to get an even treatment.

Best Red Light Therapy Device for smaller and Targeted Treatment

Bigger devices are the better but smaller devices still have the ability to treat targeted areas effectively. In facial skin treatments, smaller portable devices with sufficient power can be used to combat wrinkles and fine lines. A smaller tool can also be used to reach a problem area, such as an arthritic wrist or knee or a healing wound.

If you have a smaller, cheaper phone, make sure that you do the best. A suggested product is the Joovv Go which, like the large full-body Joovv devices, is the only portable, red light treatment system with medical strength. It is ideal for Red

Light Therapy while traveling and is the most affordable medical red light therapy available for $295.

Many near-infrared and red light therapy systems have a very small area. Most handheld devices and red lights sold online as skin enhancing devices (and many of them offer less than even this!) offer about 10mW / cm2 and only deal with a 5-10-m2 inch area, which means you would need to use the device for 30-60 minutes to cover a significant body area.

In any case, you get a gadget with a powerful output that additionally treats an enormous area at once that is where the magic is.

More powerful gadgets, similar to the lights I suggest, convey near 100mW/cm2 at around 6" from the gadget and still have compelling dosages (approximately 20-30mW/cm2) even an entire 24" away! This is an immense advantage, since now even a little light (say 15-20" long) can essentially work as if it is a full human body-sized light! As it were, an amazing light that is 15" long can be situated 24 cm or even 36 cm away from your body, and since light spreads out the more you move away from the source, that light would now be able to give a powerful portion to about your whole front or back of your body on the double! (Note: This method for utilizing it isn't perfect for profound tissues – it is perfect explicitly for hostile to maturing and skin wellbeing purposes.)

So once more, it can essentially work equivalent to a light that is multiple times the physical size (for example a light that is the size of your whole body).

Having a powerful light that is likewise huge enough in size enables you to treat enormous zones of your body without a moment's delay in only a couple of moments.

You can treat a region like the face, the entire middle or legs, or even do numerous pieces of the body and adequately, the whole body, in only a couple of moments!

High-control lights are going to give you unquestionably more advantages in far less time, are increasingly successful (particularly for profound tissues), and have greater adaptability by the way you can use them. I firmly prescribe getting a huge board light over a hand-held gadget. A great many people who buy the little gadgets end up never utilizing them since it's simply also tedious.

Power is Important, as is Independent Verification of the Device Specs

Estimating the intensity of common light is genuinely muddled, and it doesn't help that a ton of light therapy brands make huge cases about power and irradiance specs, without anything to back it up.

Here are the basics:

- *Irradiance* estimates control per unit territory, ordinarily characterized in milliwatts per square centimeter (mW/cm2). Another approach to consider irradiance is the pace of vitality delivered.

The aggregate sum of vitality delivered per territory during a light therapy treatment is measured in Joules/cm2.

- *Total Energy Matters Most:* Irradiance can be deceiving, in light of the fact that it doesn't represent how a treatment influences the individual utilizing the gadget. That is the main thing, how much all out vitality is transferred from a gadget to the individual utilizing it. All out vitality is the means by which light therapy specialists measure gadgets.

- *Ensure a Company is Legit:* Unfortunately, a large number of the cut-rate red light therapy brands make huge cases about the intensity of their little gadgets, yet don't in reality back that up with any free demonstrative information. You can't believe specs from an organization on the off chance that they haven't been autonomously tried, and you shouldn't purchase a gadget from a brand that isn't straightforward pretty much the entirety of their capacity estimations.

Bottom Line: Don't purchase a little, modest gadget that makes enormous cases about its capacity with nothing behind it. Those little gadgets won't convey anything near therapeutic evaluation red light therapy.

Modular LED Light Therapy Devices Offer the Best Design

The best red light therapy gadgets utilize particular LED gadgets to convey characteristic light over a wide surface territory of your body. They utilize this rule in a compact, handheld model that is extraordinary for focused medicines moving.

Different gadgets arrive in a wide assortment of designs, from handheld wands, to lights, to wearable belts. These gadgets are all on the least expensive finish of light therapy since they're little, under-powered, and you need to utilize them for a gigantic measure of time to get any kind of clinically-applicable advantage. A portion of these focused on gadgets might have the option to give you a couple of magnificence brings about quite certain territories, however to encounter the wide scope of advantages that originate from light therapy, you need a gadget that conveys medicinal evaluation control.

Safety First with FDA-Registered Light Therapy Devices

The immense base of clinical light therapy look into has demonstrated that regular light medications are sheltered, with for all intents and purposes, no reactions or dangers. In any case, you have to pick a quality gadget that is registered with the FDA like Joovv. Many markdown brands are not registered with the FDA, and they don't pursue GMP (Good Manufacturing Practices) either. These brands are probably going to sell you a failure gadget.

The Best Brands Offer Great Service and Help if Something Goes Wrong

You can decide the authenticity of a red light therapy organization by how much confidence they put in their items. An organization that offers a guarantee on their gadgets is significantly more liable to make a quality item than an organization that offers nothing. No guarantee is a method for saying, "when you get it, it's your concern."

Lots of things to keep an eye out for are; wavelength, the guarantee, and what precisely you need it for.

You Want Therapeutic Wavelengths that Achieve Real Results

Once more, not all wavelengths are equivalent— or all gadgets. Search for wavelengths in the demonstrated remedial reaches. In view of the majority of the examination, you need:

- 630-680nm (the ideal mending range of red light)
- 800 to 880nm (the ideal mending range of close infrared)
- Or a mix of both

What is the Warranty and How Long Will the Device Last?

This one is extremely clear – purchase from an organization with a solid guarantee who remain by their lights. Else, you'll likely be discarding cash and purchasing a substitution in a half year to a year. With an excellent red/NIR light therapy gadget from a legitimate organization, you will have it for a long-time with no issues at all. What's more, if there is an issue, they'll supplant it. In case you will burn through hundreds of dollars on something, quality is vital.

What is Your Purpose Using Red Light Therapy?

My general suggestion is that if you need to treat further tissues, organize close infrared over red light. The more you need to treat skin issues, organize red light. That is a general standard you can use to tailor your decision of a light to your remarkable needs remembering that the two kinds of light will work for most purposes. For most purposes, an enormous blended LED board with a blend of 660nm and 850nm is the best decision. Be that as it may, for explicit issues, you might need to think about different choices:

- For skin issues and male pattern baldness, it is conceivable that red light at 660nm might be the most ideal. (Despite the fact that close infrared at 850nm will even now have the greater part of similar advantages. It's only an issue of what is generally ideal.

- If you just need to treat further organ, organ, joint, or muscle/ligament issues (and NOT skin issues), at that point you might need to go with an unadulterated 850nm light gadget.

- If you just need to treat your cerebrum (for example, for despondency, uneasiness, intellectual execution, or neurological sickness), at that point close infrared is ideal. (The VieLight Neuro is likely the best choice for this particular reason).

- But for most purposes and for the vast majority, the best decision is a mix of the

660nm and 850nm LEDs in an enormous LED board that will treat a huge region of the body on the double. This choice is best since it works for fundamentally any reasons you might need it for. A joined close infrared and red light therapy gadget offering both 660nm and 850nm will enable you to do anything you need on some random day – regardless of whether hostile to maturing medications on your skin, or recuperating damage or lower back agony, or muscle recuperation and fat reduction.

My Recommended Lights for Red/NIR Light Therapy

I realize this data can feel overpowering and befuddling. So let me separate it for you basically, by giving you my top decisions for gadgets in every class from little to enormous. Here are my top decisions for the light gadgets I prescribe:

Best Medium Size Red / NIR Light Devices

These lights meet the ideal range of power supply and size, allowing large areas of your body to be handled with an appropriate dose at once. These devices generally cost up to $450 and deliver power to a large part of your body over 120-300 watts (like large muscle groups and a larger portion of the torso at a time). Similar to treating the same areas with a small device, this is a huge time saver and will result in better performance. Furthermore, because some light effects are caused by the absorption of the blood and reducing inflammation, the larger lights handle more blood at once and have greater body-wide effects. My best choices for medium-sized phones are: 1. 1. RedTherapy.co "Red Rush360."

1. *"Red Rush360" by RedTherapy.co*
   - Its 360 watts (significantly higher than the other lighting in this category) gives a robust power intensity at 6 "approximately 100mW / cm2.

- 16.3 "in height and 10.6" long (slightly larger than the other lights of this category). (That's the actual light output, not the estimated power output.)
- There are 120 LEDs (twice that of the Joovv).
- It is supplied with a 50-50 660 nm and 850 nm split.
- They have also developed new technologies for almost completely eliminating EMF emissions from their light unit, making their unit incredibly safe to use from very close distances.
- As it has very high performance, the broadest coverage, most LEDs, very competitive prices and the lowest EMFs, it is my best choice for this category.
- The price is very good for $449. (This is my overall top light option of less than $500).

2. The "BIO-300" by Platinum Therapy Lights

- 300 watts (more than twice the size of the Joovv and nearly as much as the Red Rush) gives the light a high power strength of approximately 100mW / cm2 (nearly the same as the RedRush).
- Its 19 "tall by approx 9" wide (slightly larger than the Joovv and approx. the same size as the Red Rush, not so wide a bit longer). It's got 100 LEDs.
- It is available as Joovv color, 660 nm, all in 850 nm, or a 50-50 660 nm and 850 nm split.
- The prices are very good:
- 660 nm= $449
- 50-50 split between 660
- 850 nm= $449

3. *Joovv Light "Mini" by Joovv (Joovv is the product with the longest credibility overall).*

- 120 watts, which is slightly less than the above two lights. *Note:* Their estimated power intensity is 110mW / cm2 at 6 "(6") from space, but it is based on the determined paper theoretical figures, rather than the actual light output. I measured this right next to the Platinum BIO-300 and Red Rush360 and measurements indicate that the light output is substantially lower than other devices—at ranges of 24 "or 36" away, nearly 50%.

- It's available in 660 nm (everything is 850 nm) or 50-50 nm (660 nm and 850 nm). The options for 850 nm are more costly:= $494= $560 and $460= $595= All 850 nm= $645

Best Half Body Red / NIR Light Devices

These units usually cost between $700 and $2,500 up, with a couple of great options for large, high-performance lights for under $1,000.

There are much more expensive options and complete body tools like tanning beds, which essentially treat every space of your body at once; but, for most people, they are much more expensive and unnecessary. There are many more costly red lighting "luxury" choices, but I agree that the lights in this category do not have to be surpassed. This is the category that gives you everything you need to achieve great results at a very good price. Such half-body machines are, in my experience, a fraction of the price and deliver virtually the same benefits.

Many of the devices in this section are much higher, with an output from about 300 watts at the bottom to about 600 watts.

This is great especially if paired with the opportunity to shed a lot of light on a larger area of your body at once, because the total number of photons entering the skin and the dose is dramatically increased. The results are therefore greater and the benefits are higher—especially for deeper tissue, for organ safety, muscle gain and fat losses in wider areas of your body. And per session you can do less care.

Furthermore, it is very time-efficient to treat deep tissues in large areas of your body at once, with sessions of only a few minutes, while with smaller devices it can take longer by treating several areas. So if you are looking for a large high-performance system to perform full body treatments, this is fine.

I suggest the large high-powered devices here:

1. *The BIO-600 with Platinum Therapy Lights:*

- It is 600 watts and provides a strong power strength of over 100 mW / cm2 at 6 "from the light (about twice the power output of equivalent luminaries of the other manufacturers listed below).
- It is 36 "tall by about 8" (essentially the same size as the "Original" from Joovv). (The power of Red Rush and Platinum is the same as that of the middle-size lights, but

you get it with a larger light that covers more your bodies at a time.

- It is also possible for the Joovv Original Light to be obtained in all the same choices— either 660 nm, all 850 nm or 50-50 split 660 nm and 850 nm.
- The prices are wonderful:
  660nm= $749
  $50-50 division 660= $749= $749= $749

2. *The Joovv 'Joovv Original Light'*

- Its 300 watts (about half the power output of the above-mentioned option), provides light with a power intensity of over 70mW / cm2 at 6 (Note: Again, the actual measured power density is much lower than claimed.)
• The measurements are nearly identical to those of the Platinum BIO-600.

- You can also achieve this in all the options with the Platinum light-either at 660 nm, at 850 nm, or at 5050 nm, 660 nm and 850 nm.

- Prices are significantly higher, depending on specific wavelengths you would like (around $50-$340 more): € 660 nm= $795= 50-50 fractions of 660 and 850 nm= $995= $1.0 3= $10.

3. Red Light Man's "Combo Bodylight 2.0"

- 300 watts (half the power supply of platinum light of the comparably large size and about the same as Joovv light).
- It's four feet long and about one foot longer than the other ones.
- Red and almost infrared light is used in 620 nm, 670 nm, 760 nm and 830 nm wavelengths.
- This can also be obtained as the Platinum beam, either at 660 nm, all in 850 nm, or at 50-50 splits of 660 nm and 850 nm.
- The price is $750 • It's a lovely light but, from my point of view, there are two drawbacks:

the strength isn't as powerful, particularly the platinum light.

- The portion of the light spectrum is 760 nm, which in my view isn't the ideal choice, as studies have generally shown that 700nm–780 nm wavelengths are less efficient. (This is why very few studies ever use these wavelengths.) It can still be effective, as a whole. Note: with a larger light (about 36-48) "which is so strong, you can treat the whole front or back of your body at once–even the deeper tissues. And if you'd like to do that, it's a huge investment in your wellbeing.

4. *Full Body Red / NIR Light Therapy Options*

There is also the option to make a light system that shines from the head to the middle of the whole face or back of your body.

- Joovv has a very wide 960 watt unit (the "Mega" Joovv) which is 4.5 feet in length and 16 inches in width. It comes with either pure 660 nm, pure 850 nm or a 50-50 mixture of both variants. It's an excellent light, but a lot more expensive than the above lights– you have to pay $2,400-$3,000 to get it.

- I have two Red Rush360s or Platinum BIO-300s (or one BIO-600 paired with the BIO-300 or Red Rush360s as my personal favorite set up.) I put them on my side on the floor and then sit next to them and handle one full side of my body at the same time in a position sitting instead of a position standing (which I always choose to use because I find it more comfortable to lie down compared to standing up). This light setup, as opposed to the above $2,400-$3,000 light setup, can cost less than $1,000. This is a way to get a complete body service at a very low cost.

5. *Ultra Luxury High End Red / NIR Light Therapy Options*

There are also several options available for super-high-end red-light tanning bed treatments.

These are typically over $15,000 with a well-known brand selling its device up to $100,000!

I put this in case you're interested in high-end devices (and financially you're doing well enough to make these purchases), but frankly, I really don't think those devices are needed. I do **NOT** think that the advantages of such products will be much higher than the other much cheaper lights I suggest.

The major advantage here - You can handle your entire body (front and back, head to toe) in a lying position all at once. And you may also have a pretty cool look to attract friends in your home (which might be a real consideration for certain people). Below is a list of possible entire body options:

- *Mitogen Red Light* -This consists of 10,000 LEDs that are a 660 nm and 850 nm light mixture (wavelengths identical to RedRush,

Platinum light or Joovv. The output capacity is 15mW / cm2. Treatment times are usually about 10-25 minutes.

- *NovoThor* (a well-known laser device manufacturer) also has an LED bed style full-body tanning device. This is a 630 nm, 660 nm and 850 nm mixture. It has a 17mW / cm2 power density. And it's more than $100K. This is most probably a choice for very wealthy people or for a professional gym / spa / medical environment.

Note: Such devices have relatively low power densities (less than 20mW / cm2)–possibly because they would lead easily to too many dosages if they had large power densities and handled the body as a whole at once. If this is the case, treatment times could have to be cut off at 30 or 60 seconds. Evidence also suggests that lower power densities are ideal for skin anti-aging effects and I think they would want to maximize skin benefits and systemic effects by bloodstream irradiation. These densities are, in my opinion, more suitable for anti-aging skin, but not for the treatment of deep tissue.

To be clear, I'm NOT saying or implying you have to purchase these ultra-cost phones. Nor do I suggest that red / NIR light therapy is the best way to do it. While I have learned some positive things about these light beds, I agree that with the LED lights previously recommended you can achieve all the advantage of red and near-infrared light therapy, which are small fraction of the cost of these tanned bed units.

I just mention these in order to present all the options on the market; but again, it is not to be taken as saying that you should purchase such luxurious red / nir appliances. I believe that the much less costly LED panels recommended above can provide all the benefits of Red / NIR light therapy.

Sauna + Red / NIR Light Therapy Options

There are a few sauna marks which also add close-infrared light to their sauna. It helps you to achieve all the advantages of the near infrared light discussed here while gaining the advantages (sweating, detoxification, mitochondrial advantages, etc.) of sauna water.

These are a great option if you have the cash for it, since they are much more expensive than pure red / NIR apps.

If you want something in this section, I agree that sunshine saunas are the highlights. Your mPulse sauna line contains both Far Infrared and Near Infrared. They have sauna options for 1-4 people. You can take in far-infrared + near-infrared saunas with this type of luxury sauna, and enjoy the full benefits of both near-infrared and conventional far-infrared treatment.

ClearLight Saunas also offers an excellent line of high quality far-infrared and near-infrared.

SaunaSpace produces heat lamp saunas using 4 heat lamp bulbs. The light is both far infrared and near infrared and orange. They come along with a canvas tent (as opposed to a wooden room) and are much cheaper than Sun lighten and Clarelight's wooden saunas.

This is a crucial opportunity for people who can afford it. It is also useful because it helps you to obtain your near-infrared treatment while you are enjoying a sauna.

TOP LIGHT FOR BRAIN USE

It's important to have light, not just red light, with near-infrared light—either to improve brain health or to improve mood or cognitive function. Evidence has shown that near-infrared penetrates the skull more effectively than red light (which has a minimal to no penetration of the skull), and is therefore, suitable for the brain.

The LED panel lights I recommend are almost infrared (whether pure almost infrared or mixed near-infrared with red), as the Red Rush360 and the Platinum Lights are powerful enough to penetrate the skull in light.

Nonetheless, if your main objective is to treat your brain, VieLight Neuro is the best choice, with several contact points on your head (which can be brought into contact with the scalp to allow light into the hair) and will probably produce best results for cerebrospinal problems. (Note: this device is specifically intended to be worn on the head and thus will definitely not work well to treat certain areas of the body.)

Please note that they also market intranasal devices saying that they target the brain, but Michael Hamblin, Ph.D. does not believe such devices penetrate the brain directly385, so these devices are not funded. Nevertheless, they have some good work. Hamblin claims that they don't work by radiating the brain directly, but that they work by radiating blood via the capillaries, which affect the brain (and other body systems) indirectly. If he is right, it doesn't make sense for us to use these low-power intranasal devices to treat the blood—a high-power (and far bigger) LED system would be much safer for this.

The VieLight Neuro has the head unit that is likely to target the brain effectively. So VieLight Neuro can be the best product for the specific treatment of the brain. We are not positive, because no studies compare it explicitly to LED lights, but research supports the use of this material in dementia care.

TOP 5 OVERALL LIGHTS

Here are my own suggestions for the lights that are the most dominant, financially savvy, and give astonishing blast to the buck:

1. **Red Rush360 - $449**

You can purchase this light at: https://redtherapy.co/items/redrush-360-light.
For a light this huge and amazing (360 watts) to be under $500 is simply extraordinary. It's almost multiple times the wattage of the equivalently measured Joovv, has a lot higher light yield (particularly at further separations away), and simultaneously, it costs less. It has 120 LEDs (the greater part of any light around this size, and double the quantity of LEDs as the Joovv). Generally speaking, this light is presumably perfect for a great many people's needs. Additionally, on account of its powerful thickness, you can utilize this light from 18", 24", or even 36" away and still have a sufficiently high light yield to do successful medications – subsequently enabling you to treat a

huge region of your body at the same time. Essentially, this enables it to work as a lot of bigger light. Generally speaking,, a brilliant choice for practically all reasons. I strongly prescribe it.

Furthermore, they just turned out with a line of ultra low-EMF lights! They are the main organization available. This settles on them the reasonable top-decision as I would see it as they have the most elevated power, least cost, and most minimal EMFs of any gadget in this size range.

Discount: They will give a $25 rebate to perusers of this book bringing complete expense down to $424. Simply enter the markdown code "vitality plan" when looking at.

2. *Platinum Therapy Lights BIO-600 - $789*

You can buy this light at: https://platinumtherapylights.com/products/bio-rlt. In case you are interested in an extra-huge light to basically treat the whole front or back of your body without a moment's delay, this is the light for you. In case you're hoping to go hard and fast on a bigger light without going through a huge amount of cash, this is the best approach.

Discount: They will give a $40 rebate to perusers of this book bringing all out cost down to $749. Simply enter the markdown code "vitality outline" when looking at.

3. Platinum Therapy Lights BIO-300 - $489

You can buy light at: https://platinumtherapylights.com/items/bio-rlt. This light has comparable measurements to the Red Rush360 and is nearly as amazing. It's slightly littler, yet at the same time a magnificent decision comparative with the various contenders.

Discount: They will give a $40 rebate to perusers of this book bringing all out cost down to $449. Simply enter the markdown code "vitality plan" when looking at.

4. Joovv Original - $795-$1,095

You can get this light at: https://joovv.com/items/joovv-light?variant=39356431694. This light has comparable power yield to the Red Rush360 and Platinum BIO-300 while being bigger in size (near indistinguishable measurements from the BIO-600). It is additionally extensively progressively costly, however generally, it's an extraordinary light that will enable you to treat a huge zone of your body without a moment's delay. Markdown Code: They will give a $25 rebate to perusers of this book. Utilize the markdown code "Vitality BLUEPRINT" when looking at (note: this one is case delicate, so you have to utilize all tops).

5. Joovv Mini - $495-$645

You can get this light at: https://joovv.com/items/joovv-light?variant=39356431502. This light has comparative measurements to the Red Rush360 and BIO-300, yet has altogether lower light yield (particularly at further separations away). Generally speaking, it's a great light that can unquestionably give helpful advantages, however isn't as practical as the above choices. Rebate Code: They will give a $25 markdown to perusers of this book. Utilize the markdown code "Vitality BLUEPRINT" when looking at (note: this one is case delicate, so you have to utilize all tops).

(As you can see, I have orchestrated limits for you with huge numbers of these makers offering excellent gadgets. I was not ready to orchestrate limits with the entirety of the makers recorded here; however I attempted to do it with each producer that was available to offering a rebate to perusers of this book. If it's not too much stress to know that I do get a little commission on any of these lights or saunas that you buy on the off chance that you utilize my markdown code. In case you value the work I've done recorded as a hard copy this book, I value you utilizing my markdown code. That is the way I get compensated for this work. If it's not too much trouble realize this is to no detriment to you.

Truth be told, I have arranged straightforwardly with these makers to get you limits off the typical costs by telling them that you were referred by this book. To put it plainly, everybody wins. However, if you have any issue with this, vibe allowed arranging the lights without utilizing the markdown code. If it's not too much stressful realizing that my rankings of these gadgets are not the slightest bit impacted by this. I have no proprietorship in any of these organizations or vested monetary enthusiasm for advancing any of them over another. My proposals for which light gadgets you ought to get are the very same whether you decide to utilize the rebate codes or not. Additionally, there are in reality numerous different gadgets I could advance that offer significantly more liberal commissions, which I am really not advancing in light of the fact that they don't offer great gadgets. I give you my assertion that every one of my rankings here are best on an absolutely target investigation of the power yield, quality, and value for-the-money of every one of these gadgets. My #1 need is ensuring that you get the best gadget for your needs. I have given a valiant effort to arrange the greatest limits for you as conceivable with the entirety of the producers who were available to giving limits.)

Best Sauna + Near-Infrared Options:

Sunlighten "mPulse" saunas, ClearLight "Asylum" sauna line, SaunaSpace, and SunStream Saunas (with the NIR LED board in the sauna) all offer sauna choices with both far-infrared and close infrared. For somebody hoping to get a sauna too (which likewise gives a wide assortment of astonishing medical advantages) and a red/NIR light therapy unit, these are awesome choices.

These sauna choices will in general be increasingly constrained in the manners in which that you can do the close infrared light therapy (compared with the LED gadgets), yet they make up for that disadvantage by likewise giving you the advantages of far-infrared and sauna therapy (which you don't get with red/NIR LED gadgets).

These "full range infrared" saunas are extraordinary alternatives for certain individuals, yet the cost can be an obstruction for some. If you can manage the cost of them, they're extraordinary.

Discount: I have additionally orchestrated markdown codes for you to use with Sunlighten, ClearLight, and SaunaSpace – you can call any of these organizations straightforwardly and utilize the rebate code "energyblueprint." I was not ready to mastermind a rebate code with Sunstream, however they likewise make magnificent far-infrared + close infrared saunas.

Best Brain Device:

VieLight Neuro Alpha or Neuro Gamma - $1,749

You can buy through their site here: https://vielight.com/neuro-alphagamma/

Rebate code is "vitality diagram" which gets you 10% off, which compares to $175 off the customary cost. Note: I suggest the Neuro Alpha over the Gamma.

Summarizing the Top Devices

The reasonable champs are the Red Rush360 and Platinum Therapy Lights LED boards, which essentially offer undeniably more power comparative with other comparative measured lights, and in this manner, have the additional advantage of really being lower cost than the equivalent lights in those classes.

The full-range saunas are additionally great, and the VieLight Neuro Alpha is awesome for anybody searching for mind explicit treatment.

In general, for a universally handy red/NIR light, it's difficult to beat the Red Rush360 and Platinum lights regarding the mix of by and large power and the valuing. Both of those lights is an incredible decision without anyone else – and will be consummately satisfactory for a great many people – yet if you need to go hard and fast and get a bigger light arrangement that will cover your full body, I propose getting two of the littler lights (for example two Red Rush360s or two BIO-300s), or one BIO-600. Or then again you can join a BIO-600 with either a BIO-300 or Red Rush360. (This is the thing that I for one use myself at my home.)

With these arrangements, you can get every one of the advantages of red and close infrared light therapy (that a center may charge over $100 per session for!) in the solace of your own home with boundless sessions for under $1,000 or even under $500.

CHAPTER 4

RED LIGHT DOSING

Both recommendations are based on whether the lights I suggest are available. All these numbers and formulas change if you use fewer efficient lights than I say. When you buy a different light, you will know the light intensity and calculate doses for that particular light at different distances.

- Normally 6-36 inches away from your body by the use of light.

  - Closer distances (6"-12 "from your body) are ideal for more profound treatment of the tissues.
  - Further distances from the body (12"-36) "are suitable for skin and anti-aging treatment.

- Get a strong light that can still provide an effective dose even if it is separated from your skin. In comparison to lower power lighting, it lets you handle large parts of your body at once. This is especially important for people who want to treat their skin for anti-aging purposes. I suggest that you take one of your high power lights from afar, although they are smaller (i.e., not the full size of your human body), and simultaneously manage the whole front or back of your body. Because light reaches just 15" or 20" from the source of light, when used at a further length, 40'" or 50" inches of your body can be handled at once. If you have a low-performance light and you move it a little further out of your body, the light density is out of the effective range. It makes high-performance light more cost-effective—even a little smaller with high-performance light works as a much bigger light with a far less energy and use it for its advantage!

- An ideal consumption rate from 3x-7x / week (i.e. up to once / day) is likely. (Note: There are studies which have taken more and less, but based on my experiences working with hundreds of people; I believe that it is best about three and 7 days a week.)
- Start SLOW. Do not necessarily assume that using the high end of the dose range is a good idea because "more is better." If your health is poor, start with the lowest possible doses and then increase the dosage SLOWLY. If you are extremely sick or severely exhausted, you can even start with lower doses than the lowest in my recommended range.) Also, one or two days between sessions is a great idea at first – again especially for people with bad health.
- Be careful in all sensitive dosage areas. I suggest you use only low doses of 2-10J (and perhaps lower here) if your hair, genitals or any other particularly sensitive area receive a red or near-infrared light therapy.

- We want skin problems between 3J and about 15J per area. The optimal treatment time is:
- 30 seconds to 2.5 minutes per area (6 "inches away). (But remember, if you get light I say, it'll definitely be better to go further off the skin for anti-aging skin purposes, or to take
- 1-3.5 minutes per area (if the light is 12 "away)
- 1.5-5 minutes per area (if it is 18" away). Please note that getting it away from your body will affect your body in a much bigger way at a time, because the more light spreads from the light source.
- 3–14 minutes per area — if the light is 36 "— farther away— from the body, 12" to 24' or even 36,' if the skin and anti-aging lights you would suggest are available. Remember that it can travel further with the correct light dosage for the body, but the advantage of the treatment of larger areas of the skin at once is most important.

- In comparison, they appear to be less efficient when given the Joovv light than the Red Rush360 and Platinum lights. With Joovv lights, you would like to add around 30-90% more of the above dosing ranges (especially if you use light from a larger distance from your body because of larger power differences between lights from longer distances), i.e. You might need to use the Joovv Mini for 8-12 minutes if you are 5-6 minutes away from Red Rush 360.

- In deeper matters (i.e. muscles, joints, brains, limbs, drums, fat...), we want approximately 10-40J per area, so the best treatment times and light lengths I can suggest are:
- 2-7 minutes for each area (if the light is 6" away),
- 5-10 minutes for each area (if the light is 12 "away) approximately 6" for each deeper region. You may have to take the same

dosage with the Joovv Mini for 13-15 minutes if you want to use the Red Rush360 for 10 minutes (from 12 "off).

Remember as well that some people recommend relatively higher doses for brain use (the high end of my recommended dose range), since light needs to penetrate the skin before it reaches the brain and so it is more difficult to give measurable light on the brain tissues. Thus, the brain tissue is essentially less total light (relative to fat or muscle tissue). The denser the tissue is and the more bone it is surrounded, the more fluid the target tissue requires longer doses.

- Minimum dosage / time of treatment: o I recommend that you limit to 120J the minimum therapy dose for all areas of the body. If the light is 6 "or 12" from your skin, then the light on your body shines only about 15-20 minutes of total time.

Yeah, no successful investigation is still open, so I say I'm a republican. Here's Hamblin: "What we don't know about is that your body can become overdone with total joules or is it only concentrated? That's what we do not know.... Ten or half a minute's no problem at all... Usually, I say that people can use these items for 10 or 20 minutes per day and have considerable benefits and very improbable effects.

— This would require a maximum of 12 minutes of treatment, 24J per body area and 72J for the total body dose.

- A further instance of anti-aging procedures is to treat your face 18 "for 3 minutes, your leg and thighs 3 minutes from 18," your neck and thighs 3 minutes from 18. "• Another example would be care.
- This is a maximum therapy period of 6 minutes, approximately 6J per body area, with an approximately 18J total body dose.

How to Use Your Red / Near Infrared Light System

It is possible to get confused and think using one of these lights must be terribly complex with all of these information and explanations of the science. It is not. It is not.

Yes, it's very simple and straightforward: the fundamental idea is to turn the light on and put your body before it.

All right, it's a bit more complicated, but it really isn't much more complicated. The specifics that should be known are:

1. Optimizing the tissue energy density / irradiance by changing the light range

2. Having the right dosage

3. Your position in your body

4. Practical tips / strategies for specific objectives

Let us now cover each more thoroughly.

Optimal Power Density

The general optimal power density / irradiance of the tissue you try to treat must be understood first. I will not go into this again because I already discussed the right dose in detail in the earlier paragraph. The basic idea is to use light from further afield from the body (ideally 18"-36 "away for therapy of the skin (e.g. anti-aging lamps, which I recommend) to achieve a reduced power density and a better body coverage. You want to use the light far closer to the deep tissues (6"–12 "away) to reach a high power density and to get more light into the deeper tissues.

Dose

I addressed the dose recommendations in the previous section on dosing, so refer to the time taken to use different lighting devices at different distances from your body for specific guidelines. Note that skin and surface treatments need significantly lower doses than deep tissues. And note that the overall body dose (to add all the light that is given in every area of the body you treat) is also important. See the dosing section again for all details.

Body Position

What place should you be in? You can sit, stand or sleep. Whatever is the easiest position to position yourself in relation to the light for the area of your body to be treated is the right position. Depending on what part of your body you are handling, different positions may be more relaxed than others. A hanging kit is available to hang it onto a door for many light phones, if you use it that way, you should stand (or sit in a chair) next to the phone. This is how many people do it. I use myself almost always while sleeping. I put the light on the floor and lay on my side, back or front, next to it to treat the area I am trying to deal with. Why? Why? Just because I find it more comfortable to lie down while doing it (as standing).

Practical Tips and Techniques For Specific Purposes

There are more suitable and less optimal ways to use light for specific purposes. It is the most important factor to be mindful of, because sometimes it is better to use the light in a specific way for some purposes. Yet there really isn't, for many things, any particular protocol or plan that you have to think about, so frankly, in most situations, you don't have to worry about timing or if you don't use it properly.

In most cases, you don't need to concern yourself with that, like it for oral health on your gums, reducing inflammation, wound healing or anti-aging hair, etc. Use the light on this region at any moment, when following the dosing instructions, of course.

Nevertheless, I want to discuss some aspects of how to use light to reach other objectives and how red / NIR light therapy works best with other issues. Please note that more research is necessary in the majority of cases, but from my experience and trials with hundreds of people, here are some tips:

- *Weight Loss:* Follow my plan I mentioned in the fat loss page. If you cannot do this particular morning routine, I recommend that you use it right before your workouts. You can brighten it on the fat areas you want to lose and also on the muscles you will be exercising during this training. Using light for 2-5 minutes in each area from 6 "away.
- *Removal of cellulites:* Preferably follow the previously described stubborn fat strategy, which specifically targets the light on cellulite areas of your body. Instead, if you don't do this procedure because of the timing, then just prior to exercise, use the light from the cellulite region at any time of day.
- *Immune health:* One therapy on the thymus area in the center of the chest every few days will probably support good immune health.

You can try one treatment per day during an acute infection. In the area of the thymus gland in the center of the chest I propose a treatment time of 3-5 minutes from 6'-12.

- *Anti-aging skin:* Either in the morning or in the afternoon. Use the light (if you either have a Red Rush360 or Platinum device) for 5-10 minutes from approximately 24"-36 "away. (For example, 5-10 minutes on the whole front of your body and then 5-10 minutes on your whole back.) If you are getting Joovv, the ideal range is about 24 "away (but with less wide body coverage) or 36" away for a few minutes longer (roughly twice as long) than you would have done for other lights.

- *Muscle and/or endurance enhancement:* Either right after exercise or 3-6 hours later is the ideal time for this. (Although some studies have shown muscle gains while using light prior to training). Do 3-7 minutes from a distance of 6 "in each of the muscle areas you worked on.

- *Exercise Performance:* You can use this in order to enable your muscles (endurance, strength and power) to perform better during your training. To this end, I recommend using the light on each muscle region 2-4 minutes before exercise (between 0-30 minutes before exercise).

- *Brain quality, enhanced mood (i.e. battling depression and anxiety) or brain cure:*Use the light (ideally pure almost infected light, or 50-50 combination of NIR and red, as near-infrared penetrates the skull more effectively than red light) 6"-12 "away. Since the hair blocks the sun, you want to use it without hair on a part of your face. In those with hair, it usually involves using it on the forehead or on the sides of the head, through the ear region or at the base of the neck, in comparison to getting a shaved head or being bald. The basis of your neck can target the brain fluid, which can have beneficial effects on your cells in that fluid that affect your brain's health. The front is probably the most active region and was also used in many experiments on anxiety and stimulation of the brain. As well as using the regular LED panels in this way, you can also get the VieLight neuro system, which allows you to work light into the base of your hair follicles and to provide light through the skull, even if you have skin, at various points of your face. I certainly think that it is worthwhile for people who want to concentrate on the brain as their main focus to get that VieLight Neuro unit.

- *Photopuncture:* You need a Photopuncture kit from Institute of Photonic Therapy. (Note: I don't endorse their intranasal lights, only the whole head "Neuro" device.) They provide the kit with detailed instructions on how to use the special acupuncture points "torch" light. This has been observed in particular in conjunction with tendinitis, muscle trigger point pain and migraine treatment—with very positive results.

It is also used on animals (mostly horses) by Kay Aubrey-Chimene (owner of the Photonic Therapy Institute) for many diseases and reports much success.

- *Sleep Enhancement / Melatonin Production:* As stated before certain studies suggest that red / NIR light may affect melatonin (interestingly melatonin produced by the body outside the pineal gland). Although research on the potential of red / NIR light for increased melatonin / sleep enhancement is still relatively small, I have to say that For many people, the very first time you do it is a very powerful and remarkable sleep-enhancing effect. *Here's how I recommend it:*

o Timing is key to this. Perform 1.5-2 hours before bed care. I don't advise to go to bed for less than 60 minutes.

o Using light in the spine and back of the neck for 3-7 minutes

o Caveat from about 12-18 "away. Although blue light is mainly what influences circadian rhythm and suppresses melatonin (which is usually not suppressed by red light), research has shown that high bright red light (such as Red LED Panels) can suppress melatonin. For this reason, I have several more detailed recommendations:

- I do not suggest doing so in an hour's bedtime
- I advise avoid looking into the light (that is, with your eyes closed or a towel over your face so you do not actually look into the sun).
- Also, in my experience, pure infrared lights are best used to improve sleep, because they do not have the bright red light that will

make your eyes squint. (Remember, almost infrared is invisible to most people's eyes). A simple NIR treatment on the back will make a difference in your sleep a few minutes, 1-2 hours before the night.

- *Circadian rhythm / SAD:* As already mentioned, red / NIR lights are not appropriate as SAD lights to treat / prevent seasonal psychological disorders or to improve morning rhythms with bright light. But the light systems used for the regulation of circadian rhythms / SAD prevention typically have an immense amount of blue light and little to no red or almost infrared light. Blue alone will damage both your eyes and skin so I always suggest using the red / NIR light together with the bright white / blue light to combat the black and at the same time give your cells a little healing. I suggest using the light approximately 3 feet away for this use. You may position it behind or by the bright white / blue light.

- *UV light therapy for vitamin D:* I don't mean red / NIR lights work to promote vitamin D synthesis, to be sure. You need UVb rays for that. In some cases when people live for latitudes / climates where there is little or little sunlight available during the winter months I suggest using a "vitamin D lamp," which is essentially a fluorescent bulb system that is designed specifically to emit UVb light to induce vitamin D synthesis in the body. To understand this, it is important to use the same method. In such situations, I recommend to use red / NIR light alongside UV light for the same purpose as in the circadian rhythm / SAD chapter–UV light in isolation can also damage the cells, and red / NIR helps mitigate damage and facilitates cell-healing / protection processes. For this reason, the red / NIR light can be positioned beside or behind the UV light and I recommend that the red /

NIR light from 24 "be used within 3-6 minutes to use the UV light.

- *Injuries (For example: cuts, burns, whiplash, fractures, sprains, strains, etc.):* The most important tip is in these cases to get the red / NIR light on the area as quickly as possible after initial injury. The earlier the better. I know some clinicians who claim that they have seen wounds, which normally take weeks to heal, only take a day or two because red / NIR light will arrive in the area very quickly after the injury. The other factor you have to keep in mind is whether the wound involves a surface / skin problem (e.g. slicing or burning) or a deeper problem of the tissue (e.g., bone bruise, muscle strain, sprain ligament, etc.). Implement the dosage recommendations for surface and deep tissue problems, i.e. greater ranges and higher doses of deep tissues, and larger distances and lower doses of surface tissues.

- *Treatment of fatigue / increase in energy:* For this reason, we wish to enhance the general health of Mitochondria, decrease inflammation in the blood, strengthen immune function, regulate hormones and reduce inflammation of the brain.

  - Take your clothes first and softly, and wake every cell in your body for 30-60 seconds (from 24"-36 "far away), head to head and front.

  - 1-2 minutes, roughly 6-12 "far away, on the neck and gland area and the thymus area in the middle of the head. Studies have already shown this can influence the thyroid function (studies have been done in people with the hypothyroidism of Hashimoto), which is critical for metabolic health throughout the body. The thymus light will potentially improve immune function.

- 1-2 minutes, if possible, on your sex organs, as these increases the tissue's wellbeing and facilitates optimum hormonal functioning.

- 1-2 minutes on your belly to get systemic effects by getting red / NIR light throughout your entire body's blood. Some work has shown systemic effects, likely to increase in blood radiation and blood cells, inflammatory cytokines and immune cells.

- 1–3 minutes to decrease brain inflammation and promote mitochondrial health in your brain (from 6–12), "and for a further 1-3 minutes at the base of your neck and spine.

Note: Maximum therapy time should not exceed 10-12 minutes. Be mindful that you may have to cut such doses in half or only one/4th or one or a quarter-fifth of such recommendations if you have severe fatigue (e.g. Chronic Fatigue Syndrome) or if you are extremely ill with any particular condition. Remember that the unpleasant you are the smaller doses, particularly to begin with.

CHAPTER FIVE

FREQUENTLY ASKED QUESTIONS ABOUT RED LIGHT THERAPY

Q: My specialist (chiropractor, naturopath, and so on.) said that solitary his/her laser will work and not the LED lights. Who is correct?

It is a fantasy that lone lasers have these impacts. It was thought by numerous individuals for a long time that solitary lasers had these impacts (since they were first discovered with laser gadgets), however as of late, it has been demonstrated that non-laser light (like from LED gadgets of the suitable wavelengths) have basically similar impacts.

There are more than 250 examinations utilizing LED red and close infrared light treatment that has been done in simply the most recent couple of years (since it was understood that you could get indistinguishable impacts from LEDs from lasers). The investigations that think about them have found essentially similar advantages. What's more, there is essentially nothing to demonstrate that one needs lasers to create these impacts. Indeed, even a few organizations (like Thor Laser) that have been creating laser advances for quite a long time are currently delivering LED items.

As indicated by Harvard analyst Michael Hamblin, PhD (broadly viewed as the world's top expert on close infrared and red light treatment),

"The vast majority of the early work in this field was completed with different sorts of lasers, and it was believed that laser light had some uncommon attributes not controlled by light from other light sources, for example, sunlight, fluorescent or glowing lights and now LEDs. Anyway, every one of the investigations that have been finished contrasting lasers with identical light sources with comparative wavelength and power thickness of

their discharge, have found basically no distinction between them."

Q: Are there any worries of EMFs (electromagnetic fields) if the gadget is extremely near the body?

Every electronic gadget transmit EMFs (electromagnetic fields) and the wellbeing impacts of EMFs are still discussed. By the strictest security norms from Europe, you would prefer not to normally be presented to more than 3mG (milligauss).

Only for reference for correlation, if it's not too much trouble note that your mobile phone produces considerably more than this at regular intervals, and if it's being used, radiates undeniably more than 3mG (as much as 50mG and even near 100mG). A family unit blender transmits as much as one hundred mG.

I've measured EMF yield of the Joovv, Red Rush360, and Platinum LED lights and EMF yield is moderate (keeping pace with a run of the mill PC or workstation, and not exactly a mobile phone) inside 0-3 inches. As you move away by 5 inches or something like that, there are for all intents and purposes no perceivable EMFs. (Note: EMFs drop off drastically as you move away from the source). So by utilizing it at any rate 6" away from your body, you can get a solid portion of light with no worry at all over EMFs. Anyplace over around 3" away will be exceptionally sheltered, however if you need to be amazingly wary and have no EMF introduction by any stretch of the imagination, going more than 6" is perfect. This will totally take out your presentation to EMFs. (Note: I have just figured in this reality to my suggested treatment separations illustrated in this book by encouraging you to remain in any event 6" away, so fundamentally, the EMF issue is a non-issue since there are no perceptible EMFs at the treatment separations I prescribe.)

One increasingly significant point: One should likewise consider the quality of the EMF produced, yet considerably more critically, the recurrence of the portion. What I mean is that sitting with your hands on your PC or having a cell phone on your body for a few hours every day (basic practices for a great many people in the Western world) is endlessly to a greater degree a worry for your wellbeing than a 3-or 15-minute presentation to the red/NIR light done once per day or each other day. So, in case that you're going to stress over EMFs, at that point, I propose guiding your focus toward things like the mobile phone you have on your body or in your grasp for perhaps hours every day, your utilization of PCs and iPads, and so on. Those are considerably more genuine concerns.

Also, once more, you can without much of a stretch totally take out the EMF worry with red/NIR lights out and out just by being at any rate 6 inches from the gadget. So this is actually a non-issue.

Q: What distance should the light be for most extreme impact?

The closer the light is, the more grounded the portion. So "greatest impact" would be with the LED light essentially on your body, as close as could reasonably be expected. However, in light of the fact that these electronic gadgets produce EMFs (electromagnetic fields) and the wellbeing impacts of EMFs are still discussed, I prescribe limiting EMF introduction by being at any rate 3" away from the gadget. As clarified above, going in any event 6" away is perfect.

For more profound tissues, treating from 6" or 12" is perfect. For skin and hostile to maturing impacts, there is an advantage of moving the light further-away to 12", 18", 24" or even 36", which-is that since light spreads as you move away from the source, going further away enables you to treat a lot bigger body territories at the same time.

See the dosing area of this book for progressively explicit guidelines on the best separations and portions for various purposes.

Q: How long and how frequently would it be advisable for me to do the red light sessions?

To the extent to what extent to do the treatment, this has been clarified in the area on dosing in this book. Concerning recurrence of utilization, there is no all-inclusive concurrence on the dosing recurrence in the exploration, so I can just make a suggestion dependent on what is generally regular in the examination and dependent on my encounters with a huge number of individuals I've worked with. When all is said in done, I've discovered that more than once every day is excessively. For the vast majority, the ideal recurrence is 3-6x every week. (For example: between each other day or consistently). For an intense issue, such as mending damage, it might be perfect to do one treatment for each day. (For example: You just sprained your lower leg and you need it to recuperate as quick as would be prudent). I don't suggest accomplishing more than one treatment for each day. Recollect the biphasic portion reaction clarified before in this book. Doing an excess of will give less helpful outcomes than doing the perfect sum.

Q: Is there a best time of day to do it? Or on the other hand are there sure suggested practices you have for utilizing the light for explicit issues?

There are scarcely any focuses worth making here:

- If you are utilizing the light for psychological upgrade, utilizing it on your head proceeding the period you have to center or perform is likely the best approach. (For instance in the first part of the prior day beginning your work day).
- If you are utilizing the light to improve execution during physical movement, utilize the LED on the muscles that will be most dynamic 5-an hour prior to the action.
- If you are utilizing the light to improve fat misfortune or muscle gain because of activity, utilizing it previously or after exercise is perfect (whatever season of day that is). (Note: Some investigations use it

previously and others after. I for one support utilizing it after, however there are a few examinations that have demonstrated great outcomes with applying it before practice also.)

- If you are utilizing it to speed recuperation after exercise, utilizing it directly after exercise or a few hours after the fact is perfect (whatever season of day that is).
- For most purposes – for example against maturing impacts, boosting insusceptibility and diminishing irritation – the hour of day likely doesn't make a difference by any means. (It is hypothetically conceivable that specific occasions may be slightly superior to other people, yet there is no exploration to show this).
- If you are utilizing it for cellulite reduction, it might be useful to utilize the light on the influenced territory directly before doing exercise (whatever season of day that is).

- Even however red light doesn't influence the circadian cadence so much as different wavelengths (like blue or green light, or regular indoor white house lighting, and so on.), splendid red light like these powerful LED lights will stifle melatonin discharge and upset rest on the off chance that you use it excessively near sleep time. So I would recommend not utilizing it inside an hour of rest. (NIR is likely substantially less of an issue than obvious red light in such manner).

Q: Can you split into a few little sessions for same impact?

You can conceivably do that, however I for the most part prescribe that individuals stay without any than one session for every day. I propose doing one longer treatment instead of numerous shorter medicines.

Q: I have the light and have done a few medications, however how would I realize that it's really working? How rapidly will I see or feel the impacts?

Much like enhancements or physician endorsed drugs, you can't generally realize simply dependent on your abstract sentiments if something is working or not. Take for instance a statin medicate that brings down cholesterol. Would you be able to feel that it is attempting to bring down your cholesterol? No, obviously not. In any case, that you get your blood drawn and measure your blood lipids, you will see that it is bringing down your cholesterol.

As another model, suppose you're utilizing it for muscle addition or fat misfortune, and suppose that the exploration says that as a rule, red and close infrared light treatment increment fat misfortune or muscle gain by 30% past simply doing the activity alone. (That is really an enormous impact incidentally). In any case, suppose that what that implies in pragmatic terms is the distinction between you losing 4 crawls off your abdomen (without the light) versus 5.2 inches (with the light). Except if you were estimating it and contrasting your outcomes with your indistinguishable twin doing likewise exercise and slim down arrangement as you, you have no chance to get of realizing that the light made you lose an extra 1.2 crawls of fat past what you would've lost without the light. You are absolutely ignorant of the enhancement impact of the light on your outcomes. All you know is that you got results; however, you don't have the foggiest idea how much the light added to them, since it's not as if you apply the light and watch the fat soften off just before your eyes – it's an impact that is going on gradually over weeks, and isn't something we can promptly observe or feel happening right away after the light medicines.

So much of the time, you don't generally have any method for knowing with sureness whether it is working or not simply founded on your easygoing perceptions (for example, without firmly controlling things and estimating things with versus without the light).

However, here's the uplifting news: You don't generally need to think about whether it is working, on the grounds that the genuine science has tried these things and as of now demonstrated that it works! So basically, trust the science! These researchers did unquestionably more thorough and firmly controlled investigations than you would ever do in your very own understanding, so trust their work. So this means this: Simply **DO IT**, and afterward believe that you're getting useful impacts.

Presently, there are obviously, numerous examples where one will see an impact. For instance:

- If you are utilizing it for relief from discomfort, you will see that there is a prompt torment killing impact inside 20 minutes.
- If you routinely get cut or injured here and there, and you see to what extent it normally takes you to recuperate, and afterward you

do it with the light, you will see it mends a lot quicker.

- If you are utilizing it for balding and you take photographs, you will probably see that over weeks or months, your photos show improvement.
- If you are utilizing it for joint pain, you may see following half a month or long periods of treatment that your joints hurt much less and move better, or you don't get torment the day after exercise, and so on.
- If you are utilizing it for cellulite reduction, take photographs and watch changes over a couple of months, and you'll likely observe noteworthy reduction.
- If you are utilizing it for wrinkle reduction and against maturing purposes, you will probably see impacts inside half a month (and may even have individuals praising you on how great you look)

In any case, once more, the key point is that you don't need to re-think this or marvel on the off chance that it is busy, in light of the fact that the real controlled research has just indicated that it works. So, execute what needs to be done and realize that you are accomplishing something which science has just demonstrated works. Trust the science, and do what needs to be done! :)

Q: How would we be able to be certain we are duplicating the conditions in the investigations and what specifically are the key focuses we should be aware of during our sessions?

My suggested dosing ranges in this book depend on the exploration. These general dosing rules depend on the main part of the information. So by following these dosing rules for your particular issues, you'll be in accordance with the exploration. Basically, that is actually all you have to know, so don't over think it to an extreme.

Q: What are the general advantages of 660nm (red light) and 850nm (NIR) and the upsides and downsides of joining these in one unit?

As clarified already, red and close infrared act through a similar component. The significant contrast is the infiltration profundity. Be that as it may, see the past segment on red versus close infrared for a progressively nitty-gritty talk of the distinctions.

Since both red and close infrared work through similar systems, there truly are no all-inclusive upsides and downsides – it's subject to how you need to utilize it. In case you need to utilize it to treat further tissues like organs, muscles, or the mind, go for unadulterated close infrared or a 50-50 blend. If you need to do hostile to maturing or mend things more in the surface tissues, red light may have a preferred position. In any case, if it's not too much trouble remembers that BOTH red light and approach infrared will work for the two purposes. At the point when we talk about these distinctions, it's simply a question of degrees of adequacy, not excessively one works for a particular reason and the other doesn't work by any means. The two of them work for basically these reasons, so don't over think it, and persuade yourself that the red light won't work for treating muscles, organs, and so forth. The one exemption may be, where it has been demonstrated that close infrared enters much preferable through the skull over unmistakable red light does. Then, in case you need to utilize it to improve mind wellbeing, close infrared is a superior decision,

Q: What is the hazard to eyes? Any risk after waterfall medical procedure? How best to secure the eyes as a pre-alert? Any contrasts between red versus close infrared here?

When all is said in done, the examination demonstrates that red and close infrared light are very valuable for eye wellbeing. While there is no official accord among analysts about this, I think all things considered, you needn't bother with any extraordinary defensive eyewear as you would with numerous different kinds of light, similar to UV light. , there is some exploration showing that long-span presentation in the eyes may not be a smart thought, and you might need to keep the portion extremely low for the eyes (for example, the eyes may not endure bigger dosages just as other body parts.) One scientist remarked:

"Eye security: In an investigation by Merry et al (2016), 50-80 mW/cm2 of obvious red light appeared to improve vision, however in that review, subjects kept their eyes shut while taking a gander at the Warp10 treatment gadget (670nm). Another logical article on eye wellbeing expressed that 10 mW/cm2 would be a protected furthest breaking point for a close infrared presentation of long span."

If you have a particular condition or eye medical problem (for example post waterfall medical procedure), if you don't mind converse with your primary care physician and ensure it's alright for you.

I will likewise make reference to, significantly, that lasers are altogether different from LEDs. You ought to NEVER sparkle lasers at you!

However, LEDs are a lot more secure for light presentation in the eyes. Regardless of whether they are 100% impeccably ok for huge dosages isn't yet thoroughly clear. In case you have any eye medical issues and you need to decide in favor of alert, you may need to:

1. Make sure that you just open your eyes to low portions (under 5 Joules is most likely a decent gauge). For example, substantially less than you would portion the various territories of your body.

2. Close your eyes or wear texture (for example towel, shirt, blindfold, and so forth.) around your eyes while utilizing the light.

Until we have increasingly definitive information, it doesn't damage to decide in favor of alert.

(Once more, counsel your PCP if you have a particular issues – these announcements are not planned as medicinal guidance or cases to treat or fix a particular eye condition).

The one other contrast here is basically eye affectability. A few people discover the splendor of an incredible red LED light to be challenging for the eyes (as in any splendid light will be). So if you are delicate to the light, don't hesitate to close your eyes or utilize a type of texture or blindfold to cover your eyes. Note that the close infrared light isn't obvious to the human eye, so you won't have any brilliant light that your eyes are touchy to with close infrared.

Q: What on the off chance that you have certain tricky tissues like tumors or growths? Are there any hazard factors when sparkling it over a territory where one has polycystic ovaries or maybe a benevolent sore on a bosom and so on? Should these zones be covered when treating?

(Standard disclaimer: For a particular ailment, if you don't mind counsel your PCP before utilizing red or close infrared light. Nothing I state here ought to be translated as medicinal guidance or as a case to treat or fix any condition.)

When all is said in done, red and close infrared light will be animating to tissues that you sparkle it on, so it is sensible to guess (despite the fact that we don't have a lot of information to go on) that sparkling it on carcinogenic tumors would most likely not be a smart thought. Despite the fact that Michael Hamblin said that by and large, the examination shows improved results in malignant growth when red/NIR light is utilized on OTHER PARTS of the body (for example not simply the tumor).

With respect to growths or polycystic ovaries, there is actually no exploration on this. In any case, as a prudent guideline, I would recommend not sparkling it on any tissues that you would prefer not to conceivably invigorate.

I accept that I am by and large exorbitantly careful in my suggestions here, yet I believe it's keen to do as such until we have more research to put together proposals with respect to.

Q: Will it assist decline with fatting and cellulite and how can it help do as such? Is it just by the method for losing fat or simply by sparkling on territory of skin?

To the extent cellulite is concerned, it reduces cellulite fundamentally by improving the auxiliary respectability of the collagen systems. (It likewise may work by invigorating fat misfortune).

For fat misfortune, red/NIR light without anyone else's input (for example, without nourishment and way of life mediations) likely won't do a lot to assist you with losing fat. (Although examination proposes it may even now support a piece). Where it's truly going to sparkle is if you are really occupied with sustenance and way of life schedule that is generally driving fat misfortune. In that situation, it will enhance the impacts and enable you to lose much progressively fat. Be that as it may, once more, independent from anyone else, simply doing the red/NIR light without nourishment and way of life transforms, you won't see a lot of advantage on fat misfortune. It is anything but an enchantment pill, yet rather a key way of life system that intensifies the advantages of another way of life methodologies.

Q: What makes the red light restorative – is it the measure of nm? I found an alternate light that is 660nm and it's just $50 or $100 or $150. Do I truly need to get the ones that are $400 and up?

It's not simply the wavelength that issues. For instance, I can give you a little LED gadget with 10 bulbs of 3 watts every that is a 660nm gadget and it may just cost $14, yet it's essentially useless on the grounds that it's way too underpowered, and it won't enlighten a critical part of your body.

The portion (intensity of the light joined with the good ways from your body), alongside being a sizable light, alongside being at the correct wavelength are on the whole key elements.

Any light that you've discovered that is modest is more likely than not missing at least one of those three components

Should you don't have a light that can give a compelling portion to your body (and the perfect measure of your body), you have a gadget that is for the most part useless.

Believe me, it is a HUGE slip-up not to tune in to my recommendation in this book about getting a gadget with satisfactory power. You can get a portion of the gadgets available that are 30 watts or 60 watts for $100 or $300 or $400, yet you will have quite recently squandered your cash, in light of the fact that those gadgets can't give you a viable portion. So don't purchase the less expensive gadgets, and set aside your cash to get one of the gadgets from the brands I am prescribing here. It's the distinction between getting results and not getting results.

What's more, recollect that these gadgets I prescribe that are $449-$1,000 dollars are quite modest compared to getting a laser ($5,000-$30,000) or heading off to a center to get medicines ($75+ per treatment).

Q: I am confounded by all these various terms like photobiomodulation (PBM) and Low-Level Laser Therapy (LLLT). What are these and how would they contrast from red/NIR light treatment?

To put it plainly, these are for the most part essentially tradable terms. So don't get befuddled by cites or different individuals who use terms like "photobiomodulation" or LLLT? Indeed "LLLT" itself doesn't constantly mean something very similar – a few people compose it as "low-level laser treatment" and others as "low-level light treatment."

Generally, it was believed that lasers (intelligent light shafts) had one of kind impacts that were entirely unexpected from standard wellsprings of light like lights or LEDs. Accordingly, the main part of the exploration has been finished with lasers and utilizations the expression "low-level laser treatment" or LLLT for short.

To make things much progressively muddled, numerous different terms have been placed into utilization by certain individuals like "cold laser," "restorative laser," "photobiotherapy," and so forth.

(*Side note:* There is additionally the wide term "light treatment" which individuals use to mean a wide range of things inconsequential to red/NIR light treatment, similar to treatment for the eyes, or rest issues, or utilizing a SAD light for occasional full of feeling issue, and different employments.)

In any case, back to red and close infrared light treatment...

Lately, it has become acknowledged that lasers don't have the one of a kind impacts once thought, and that it's simply light at these wavelengths in the correct power (not explicitly laser pillars) that produce these impacts.

So now there have been hundreds of concentrates on red/NIR light treatment that utilization ordinary LED boards (not lasers). This is at times, referred to explicitly as LEDT (LED treatment) or all the more extensively as still LLLT, yet now characterized as "low-level light treatment" (instead of laser treatment).

Since it has been discovered that it's not just lasers that produce these impacts, most specialists presently utilize the wide and sweeping terms "low-level light treatment" (still with LLLT) or the better term, "photobiomodulation" (which implies actually the changing of science with light).

But, once more, don't get befuddled by these various terms. For our motivations here, these terms are inter-changeable with "red and close infrared light treatment."

Q: Do red light gadgets discharge UV light?

No, they don't. UV light is another piece of the light range altogether separate from red and close infrared. The light gadgets I prescribe don't radiate any UV light.

Q: Can I utilize any red light to get the advantages?

No. As I clarified in the area on picking a gadget, you need a gadget that has enough power (wattage), is of good size for what you need to utilize it for, and has the best possible wavelengths of light.

Q: Does red light treatment tan you or consume the skin?

No. Tanning and sun copies originate from UV beams. These gadgets don't discharge UV light.

Q: Do you get Vitamin D from red light?

No. Our body orchestrates nutrient D from introduction to UV-b light. These gadgets don't emanate UV light.

In case you are hoping to orchestrate nutrient D, you need introduction to either sunlight or a strength UV light (I propose the Sperti UV-b light for this reason.

Q: Can I get the advantages of red/NIR light treatment by remaining in the sun?

Truly and no. It's somewhat of a nuanced answer...

To start with, in all actuality if you were going through hours consistently outside with the sun on your skin (like our precursors did), at that point you most likely needn't bother with a red/NIR light gadget.

In any case, since a large portion of us don't go through hours daily with the sun on our body, we end up inadequate in the supplement of red/NIR light. So getting a red/NIR light gadget is an exceptionally shrewd move.

I should make reference to that the sun has benefits that red/NIR light gadgets don't have. The sun emanates UV light, which we use for a few purposes, such as integrating nutrient D. It's additionally going to be better for setting circadian mood toward the beginning of the day.

In any case, red/NIR lights additionally have a few focal points over the sun...

One is comfort and access. Not every person lives in a spot that is radiant lasting through the year. What's more, not every person can get outside in the sun each day during the hour of day where it's warm and radiant (and you'd need to have your skin uncovered.)

What's more, for much focused on medications of explicit issues, the sun won't give you the accuracy focusing of a light gadget. That is, you can sparkle a light gadget explicitly on the thyroid organ or on a particular injury site with the exact light power and portion that will prompt the best impacts.

Additionally, the range contrasts in significant ways that influence a few objectives. Specifically, for the skin against maturing (on the face for instance), numerous individuals would need to abstain from getting loads of UV all over from the sun (which may quicken skin harm and skin maturing), yet get the advantages of red/NIR. The sun doesn't enable you to do this – with the sun, and you get the entire range of red, close infrared, far-infrared, blue, and UV. Be that as it may, with a red/NIR light gadget, you can get the restorative advantages on your skin while staying away from the possibly counterproductive wavelengths altogether.

Honestly, red/NIR light gadgets are not a trade for sunlight. Despite everything we need a lot of sun introduction to be sound. Yet, red/NIR light gadgets can compensate for our absence of sun presentation and give us a few focused on benefits such that we can't get from the sun.

Q: I see a few people utilizing blue lights in their gadgets, what are the contrasts among blue and red lights?

These organizations that do this are confused, as I would like to think. Blue light doesn't have indistinguishable physiological impacts from red/NIR light, and actually, has a few impacts which contradict red/NIR light.

All things considered, blue light is fundamental and crucial to our wellbeing since blue light entering our eyes encourages into our circadian musicality/check in mind, which manages various hormones and synapses, and numerous essential capacities. So I am not saying that blue light is awful – in actuality, we need blue light to be solid (particularly blue light entering our eyes). (Note: There are additionally some other potential employments of blue light like brightening teeth or treating skin inflammation.)

In any case, blue light straightforwardly on the skin, or on wound/damage locales, muscle tissue (or anything where one may utilize red/NIR light) is an impractical notion. The blue light isn't doing anything gainful all things considered, and may even be cheapening the advantages of red/NIR light. Explicitly on account of hostile to maturing medicines on the skin, it is nearly destined to be counter-gainful, as blue light can harm the skin cells.

In addition, we as a whole invest gigantic measures of energy inside under fluorescent or LED indoor lights that have huge amounts of blue light. Our own gadgets like telephones, PCs, ipads, and so forth additionally radiate heaps of blue light.

So a large portion of us are being washed in blue light constantly, and we're hugely lacking in red/NIR. Once more, blue light doesn't invigorate indistinguishable physiological advantages from red/NIR light.

Q: Does red/NIR light treatment work through garments?

The short answer is no. In case that the garments are extremely thin and light can enter it well, at that point perhaps somewhat. How would you know whether red light can infiltrate it? Just hold the texture up alongside the light while it's on, and perceive how much light gets past. You can actually watch it with your unaided eye.

Presently, with most garments, they will hinder in any event half and increasingly like 80%+ of the light, so if that is the situation, simply understand that it is enormously bringing down the portion of the light.

To summarize: I wouldn't prescribe attempting to do any light medicines through attire. For best outcomes, do it on exposed skin.

Q: What is the distinction between these red/NIR light gadgets and plant develops lights that some plant producers use, or lights on coral reef aquariums?

Plant developing lights and coral developing lights use lights with a wide range of parts of the range – blue, UV, green, red, orange, and so on. (There are a couple of plant develop lights that are simply red, yet they are for the most part incredibly underpowered, and don't have ideal pillar edges.)

Red and close infrared lights use LEDs that explicitly produce just red as well as close infrared light at the particular restorative wavelengths, and at the correct power yield for remedial impacts. However, the short answer is no, you can't utilize plant developing lights or aquarium

Lights as red/NIR light treatment gadgets. They are entirely unexpected. If you need to do red/NIR light treatment, get the correct sort of light gadget explicitly intended for that reason.

Q: Can it be utilized while pregnant?

There is no information on this, so we can't state without a doubt. I will say that people get red/NIR light introduction from the sun (for example so this happens constantly – at whatever point a pregnant lady is sunbathing). In any case, it is practical that red/NIR gadgets could vary somehow or another that has sudden impacts. Hence, since we don't have the information on this, I will stay with my prudent proposals similarly as with the above remarks, and encourage you to decide in favor of alert and don't do anything which we don't have a clue about the impacts of.

Be that as it may, once more, counsel your primary care physician first and consistently decide in favor of alert

Q: Can you explain measurements on a specific territory of the body compared to add up to session dose? As such, if max measurements is 20 mins would i be able to complete 20 mins on every zone or 20 minutes max for all territories joined (for example if 2 territories 10 mins each)?

Max dose is the most extreme absolute treatment time for all regions treated. That implies that you can either complete 20 minutes (conceivably) on one zone of the body, or separation that 20 minutes over various zones. It doesn't mean 20 minutes on every territory.

Note: 20 minutes is the most extreme measurement (in view of the lights I am encouraging you to get). What's more, recall that doing the greatest isn't really the best. A great many people will see preferred impacts with lower portions over the most extreme dosages in the suggested dosing range. What's more, particularly individuals who are in exceptionally unexpected frailty should begin with a lot littler dosages at the extremely base (or underneath) the prescribed dosing range.

If you do a more extended treatment time like 15-20 minutes, I unequivocally recommend doing it on more than one zone of the body (for example 2-4 zones), instead of the entire 20 minutes just on one territory. 20 minutes on one zone will very likely be excessively solid of a portion on that territory of the body.

- *Total Treatment Dose/Time:* To figure the absolute portion all the more unequivocally, if it's not too much trouble, see the prior segments that went over on control thickness numbers (for example, 100mW/cm2) and how that identifies with the measure of Joules. I propose that you limit the absolute treatment portion for all zones of the body that ought to be close to generally 120J. So accepting the light is 6" or 12" away from your body. That implies close to about 15-20 all-out minutes of time with the light sparkling on your body.

Q: If you have peculiar and serious vision impacts after your eyes are presented to either the red or close infrared LED lights, how might you decide whether it is as yet safe to uncover your eyes?

When in doubt, on the off chance that you notice any negative impact, bring down the portion. To the extent this enhanced visualization explicitly, first, it's genuinely ordinary to see spots in the wake of being presented to any splendid light. On the off chance that you feel your vision is altered in some significant manner or you don't care for any special visualizations that it causes, don't hesitate to cover your eyes (or straightforward close them) while utilizing the light.

Q: You gave critical extents for treatment times, so how would I know whether I ought to accomplish for instance, brief versus 10 minutes?

There is no all-inclusive method for dosing here, in light of the fact that it varies between people. On the off chance that you are in unexpected frailty or are seriously exhausted, I generally suggest beginning with littler dosages, and a few people in extremely unforeseen weakness can feel exhausted from doing excessively (similarly that they may from over working out). So in the initial barely any medicines use times at the lower end of my suggested dosages. If you ever feel exhausted subsequent to utilizing it that implies you overcompensated the portion. So lower the portion on your next session.

To make it straightforward: I propose beginning with littler dosages, and afterward working up to the higher parts of the bargains treatment times through the span of half a month. At that point, on the off chance that you ever feel exhausted, back off the portion a piece and you've discovered your optimal portion, or on the other hand don't hesitate to keep utilizing the portions at the higher finish of my suggested dosages if you have no antagonistic response to it and you feel great from it (as most sound individuals will).

Q: Can you clarify the distinction between the LED lights accessible to the overall population and the more costly laser gadgets just accessible to therapeutic experts? Is there strong research to show that they have similar impacts? How would you decide the parameters of treatment utilizing a LED gadget that would be practically identical to the parameters of treatment utilized in an examination utilizing a Laser gadget?

Truly, there is a lot of research to show that they have equivalent impacts. What's more, if it's not too much trouble see the statement from the world's first master regarding this matter, Michael Hamblin, PhD, prior in this book where he unequivocally says that they have essentially similar impacts. It is additionally significant that he himself utilizes a LED gadget, not a laser gadget. (He utilizes it on his brow in the mornings to improve cerebrum/intellectual capacity).

To the extent the parameters of treatment utilizing a laser versus a LED gadget, you do this by ascertaining the all-out portion they utilized and utilizing a similar portion with the LED. (Keep in mind; it's only a component of all-out vitality delivered, so it tends to be determined with a laser or LED gadget fine and dandy.) To disentangle this (and make it so you don't feel that you have to do complex computations to make sense of this), simply pursue my dosing rules.

Q: When utilizing it for the mind, are there large contrasts between red versus close infrared light? What's more, does the light enter through hair, and through the skull?

NIR will overcome the skull all the more viably, so for the mind explicitly, close infrared will be unrivaled.

Neither close infrared nor red light will infiltrate viably through hair, so you would prefer not to sparkle it on the bushy pieces of your head, however the temple, back of the neck, and ear territories are altogether great.

Additionally, it's important that specific gadgets are intended to focus on the cerebrum explicitly. VieLight is an organization that makes mind explicit gadgets. They sell intranasal gadgets that are professed to focus on the cerebrum. Yet, Michael Hamblin, Ph.D. doesn't accept these gadgets really arrive at the mind straightforwardly, but instead they work through lighting the blood in the vessels, which by implication influences the mind (and different frameworks of the body). Expecting that he is right, it truly doesn't bode well to utilize these low-control intranasal gadgets to treat the blood – it would be greatly improved to utilize a high power (and a lot bigger) LED gadget for that reason.

, VieLight additionally makes an item called VieLight Neuro which is a lot higher power gadget with different light focuses around the skull. (It tends to be put to produce light through the hair follicles legitimately on the skin, so the hair doesn't hinder the light). What's more, the VieLight Neuro might just be the best item for treating the cerebrum explicitly. We don't know without a doubt, as there are no examinations contrasting it with LED lights, yet it seems to be an incredible item.

Q: Are there any suggestions on the best way to utilize the light contrastingly during the various seasons?

This is an intriguing inquiry. We don't have any information on this, so my answer will be theoretical. With UV lights, we realize this is truly clear: Obviously you use UV light on your skin to help integrate more nutrient D during the time where you get less sun – the winter. On account of red/NIR light, we are not worried about nutrient D explicitly, yet I would state pursue a similar standard of doing significantly more in the winter (likewise with utilizing an UV light) to compensate for absence of sun introduction in winter. This is particularly valid for any individual who lives in a spot where they don't get a lot of sun introduction throughout the winter months.

Q: Are there any reactions of utilizing a red/NIR light gadget? Would you be able to do excessively?

Recollect that red/NIR light has a "biphasic portion reaction" (we discussed this prior in the book). That implies that at exceptionally low portions, you will get practically zero impact. At the correct portion, you'll get great impacts. Furthermore, if you do substantially more than that, you will return to having next to zero impact. So kindly pursue the prescribed dosing rules, and know that accomplishing more than that will prompt less outcomes as opposed to more outcomes.

To the extent explicit reactions, much of the time for the vast majority, there is almost no danger of symptoms. The fundamental concern is essentially doing too enormous of a portion, in which case, you would chiefly just not get benefits instead of cause some horrible reactions.

As opposed to state, utilization of UV light (for example tanning beds) — where there is an enormous danger of cell harm by trying too hard — red/NIR light is uncommonly protected and has little danger of negative reactions

, a little level of individuals will encounter reactions from doing excessively. The fundamental symptoms are cerebral pains and weariness/depletion (since it can require a lot of vitality to manage the mending and mitochondria-animating properties of red/NIR light).

Likewise potential side effects are from the EMFs from the gadget. A few people are very delicate to EMFs (you know whether you are, on the grounds that your mobile phone and workstation/tablet cause significant side effects for you). Similarly, the EMFs from a light can be tricky if you choose to put the light gadget directly on your body and don't leave a few crawls of room between your body and the light. (See my proposals on keeping the light at any rate 3" away, and I'd recommend in any event 6" for any individual who is EMF delicate. At 6" there will be next to zero distinguishable EMFs).

Another potential symptom is poor rest in the individuals who utilize the light just before sleep time. This is on the grounds that despite the fact that red colored light doesn't for the most part stifle melatonin creation (melatonin is vital for good rest), if the light is sufficiently high force/control, it in reality still will smother melatonin – much like light from your TV or wireless will. This is the reason it's best not to utilize the light inside an hour of sleep time.

One more thing worth referencing here is that sure individuals appear to be unquestionably more touchy than others with the impacts of red/NIR light. What's more, the portion that is ideal for one individual might be far lower than someone else. When all is said in done, I've discovered that individuals with serious medical issues are here and there extremely delicate with the impacts of the light and need MUCH lower portions. A few people in this circumstance may encounter weariness/depletion or cerebral pains even from generally low dosages. This is likely because of the distinctions in by and large redox balance in cells. In particular, individuals in unforeseen weakness or those with different constant sicknesses may have very raised degrees of oxidative pressure (abundance free radicals) in their body, and the hermetic impacts of things like exercise or red light treatment might be intense for their cells to deal with. So similarly as over-practicing can cause weariness/weakness in these individuals, so too can exaggerating the red/NIR light treatment.

The answer for this is generally straightforward: If you are in unexpected frailty or are seriously exhausted, I generally suggest beginning with littler dosages. So in the initial not many medicines, use times at the low finish of (or underneath) my prescribed portions. At that point gradually increment the portion on ensuing treatment sessions (inside my suggested portion extend) to locate your maximal portion underneath the edge of any reactions. If you ever feel exhausted in the wake of utilizing it that implies you overcompensated the portion. So lower the portion on your next session.

CONCLUSION

Red light treatment/LLLT (low-level laser treatment) is a protected, synthetic-free, torment free system that is well-endured with no hurtful symptoms. By emanating red, low-light wavelengths through the skin to animate cell revival, increment bloodstream, invigorate collagen and that's only the tip of the iceberg; red light treatment has indicated a critical potential for improving our wellbeing and prosperity. It offers patients an unwinding, non-equivocal experience that has rapidly turned into a prominent option in contrast to customary medications on account of its application and advantages.

Red Light treatment/LLLT medications have various advantages from recuperating wounds, reducing torment and fixing tissue, improving joint and muscle wellbeing to treating the reactions malignancy patients experience from chemotherapy and radiation. Red light treatment has become a progressive treatment for hostile to maturing and male pattern baldness.

Clinical and logical proof for red light treatment unquestionably appears to be persuading... and, promising. However, many are still somewhat doubtful about the level of adequacy red light treatment produces. What's more, on the grounds that the employment of new medications relies upon FDA endorsement in the western universe of medication, numerous specialists and scientists concur further research is required.

Made in the USA
Las Vegas, NV
24 January 2023